Yoga Games
for Children

Other SmartFun Books

101 Music Games for Children by Jerry Storms

101 More Music Games for Children by Jerry Storms

101 Drama Games for Children by Paul Rooyackers

101 More Drama Games for Children by Paul Rooyackers

101 Dance Games for Children by Paul Rooyackers

101 More Dance Games for Children by Paul Rooyackers

101 Movement Games for Children by Huberta Wiertsema

101 Language Games for Children by Paul Rooyackers

Coming Soon

101 Improv Games for Children and Adults by Bob Bedore

Ordering

Trade bookstores in the U.S. and Canada, please contact:

Publishers Group West
1700 Fourth Street, Berkeley CA 94710
Phone: (800) 788-3123   Fax: (510) 528-3444

Hunter House books are available at bulk discounts for course adoptions;
to qualifying community, health-care, and government organizations;
and for special promotions and fund-raising. For details please contact:

Special Sales Department
Hunter House Inc., PO Box 2914, Alameda CA 94501-0914
Phone: (510) 865-5282   Fax: (510) 865-4295
E-mail: sales@hunterhouse.com

Individuals can order our books from most bookstores,
by calling toll-free **(800) 266-5592**, or from our
website at **www.hunterhouse.com**

Yoga Games

Children

Fun and Fitness with Postures,
Movements, and Breath

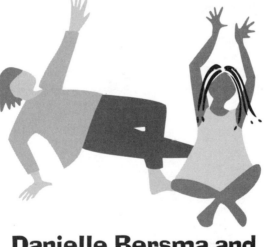

Danielle Bersma and
Marjoke Visscher

Translated by Amina Marix Evans &
Illustrated by Alex Kooistra

a Hunter House *SmartFun* book

First published in the Netherlands in 1994 by Panta Rhei as
Spelen Met Yoga

Hunter House Inc., Publishers
PO Box 2914
Alameda CA 94501-0914

Library of Congress Cataloging-in-Publication Data

Bersma, Danielle.
    [Spelen met yoga. English]
    Yoga games for children : fun and fitness with postures, movements, and
breath / by Danielle Bersma and Marjoke Visscher ; translated by Amina Marix
Evans.
        p. cm. — (A Hunter House smartfun book)
    Includes index.
    ISBN 0-89793-390-7 (spiral) — ISBN 0-89793-389-3 (pbk.)
    1. Yoga, Haòha, for children. 2. Exercise for children. I. Visscher,
Marjoke. II. Title. III. Series.

RA781.7 .B4713 2002
613.7'046—dc21   2002075931

Project Credits

Cover Design and Book Production:
  Jil Weil

Book Design: Hunter House

Developmental & Copy Editor:
  Ashley Chase

Proofreader: John David Marion

Acquisitions Editor: Jeanne Brondino

Editor: Alexandra Mummery

Editorial & Production Intern:
  Claire Reilly-Shapiro

Publicity Coordinator:
  Earlita K. Chenault

Sales & Marketing Coordinator:
  Jo Anne Retzlaff

Customer Service Manager:
  Christina Sverdrup

Order Fulfillment: Lakdhon Lama

Administrator: Theresa Nelson

Computer Support: Peter Eichelberger

Publisher: Kiran S. Rana

Printed and Bound by Bang Printing, Brainerd, Minnesota

Manufactured in the United States of America

9 8 7 6 5 4 3 2 1   First Edition   03 04 05 06 07

Contents

*A detailed list of the games indicating
appropriate age groups begins on the next page.*

List of Games

List of Games, continued

List of Games, continued

Lessons with a Theme

Preface

Children are natural yogis. Watch children at play, and you will see them spontaneously strike poses that often happen to be traditional *yoga asanas,* such as downward dog, the child's pose, and the plow. They also invent their own unique poses. Some yoga poses are not suitable for children's growing bodies, but the general practice of yoga does not have to be watered down for kids. The practice of yoga is a growth process in which each phase is as important as the next.

This book is written for yoga teachers, activity-group leaders, elementary-school teachers, and parents who are looking for fun ways to exercise with their children. These games are ideally suited for yoga classes in a school, camp, community center, or workshop setting. They are also useful for physical education, dance, and drama classes. In addition, short yoga exercises can serve as a welcome break or pick-me-up in a homeroom class setting. With slight adaptation, many of the exercises can be done while sitting at a desk. Taking a moment to breathe, relax, or stretch will leave students calm and alert, ready to learn. (See "Yoga in the Classroom" on page 6.)

The games are explained in a simple and straightforward manner. Although yoga brings a sense of awareness to the games, they also involve healthy doses of fun and pleasure.

We wrote this book because we love children, we were once children ourselves, we gave birth to children, and we work with children. The child, with all her possibilities and limitations, is at the center of this book.

Danielle Bersma and Marjoke Visscher
The Netherlands

For easy reading, we have alternated use of the male and female pronouns. Of course, every "he" also means "she," and vice versa.

Becoming a child

with children

sharing the wonder

sharing imagination

being a child

makes you complete

Important Note

The material in this book is intended to provide information about a safe, enjoyable exercise program for children. Every effort has been made to provide accurate and dependable information. The contents of this book have been compiled through professional research and in consultation with professionals. However, professionals have differing opinions, and some of the information may become outdated; therefore, the publisher, authors, editors, and professionals quoted in the book cannot be held responsible for any error, omission, or dated material. The authors and publisher assume no responsibility for any outcome of applying the information in this book. It should also be noted that children's bodies are fragile, so they should not be forced to adopt any physical positions that cause them pain or discomfort. If you have questions concerning your exercise program or about the application of the information described in this book, consult a qualified professional.

Introduction

Objectives of the Yoga Games

As the saying goes, children need two things from us: roots and wings. Children need a protective, loving, and secure environment to grow into healthy adulthood. Only when they have put down roots and become grounded in the earth can they develop wings that will carry them freely through life. The aim of this book is to make a contribution to this process—to increase children's self-awareness and self-confidence through breathing and movement. In their modest way, these yoga games are designed to help children feel grounded, develop a firm stance, and find their balance—and then begin exploring flight.

The games serve various educational goals applicable to yoga, physical education, dance, and drama classes. They are also valuable to players' personal and social development. The games are designed to:

- **improve motor skills and physical fitness**
  The various poses and movements involved in the yoga games develop children's flexibility, strength, balance, and posture. The breathing exercises teach children to breathe properly and expand their lung capacity, increasing endurance. The relaxation games help children understand not only how to exercise their bodies, but how to relax them. You will find that these games help balance children's energy levels—after a yoga session, children who are extremely active will be calm and relaxed, while quiet children will become more alert. Finally, many of the games give children a better understanding of how their bodies work and move.

- **develop awareness of the senses**
  These games help children to become more observant. Different games encourage them to use their senses of sight, hearing, smell, taste, and especially touch. By helping children notice sensory input that they might have overlooked otherwise, these games give children a new perspective on the world around them, each other, and themselves.

- **foster emotional growth**
  Physical well-being enhances mental well-being. Yoga addresses the person as a whole: Mind and body are one. The yoga games help children balance their emotions, relax their minds, strengthen their concentration, and be flexible when met with unexpected circumstances.

  Through meditation exercises (sitting still) the older child will learn to observe his thoughts and to realize that there is more to him than just "I'm pretty; I'm ugly; I'm scared; I'm stupid; I'm the greatest." Children can discover their feelings and learn to enjoy themselves. And us? We can discover and enjoy the children.

- **build social skills**
  The games in this book give players ample opportunities to work in pairs, in small groups, and as a class. Several of the poses and movements will not work unless two or more children cooperate. Children come to appreciate the fact that they can sometimes achieve more through working together than they can on their own. Doing exercises together stimulates the children's ability to negotiate with and pay attention to each other, thus making them more considerate of others. In many games, children are invited to invent poses and movements and display them to each other. This helps them gain self-confidence. In addition, the book includes a series of trust games to help players develop mutual faith and respect. The children learn how to work with others in a group while retaining their own individuality.

- **foster creativity**
  Various games give children opportunities to improvise movements, engage in fantasy play, make drawings, and otherwise

express themselves creatively. The games encourage children to maintain their spontaneity and originality, and to carry these forward into their later lives.

Children and Yoga

Which yoga poses are suitable for a child and which are not? To answer this question, we must first consider the question: What is a child? Children are very different at different stages of development. The games in this book are all labeled with icons that tell at a glance the recommended age group. (See "Key to the Icons Used in the Games" on page 12.) In this way, you can choose games that support children's different levels of maturity and motor skills. Children who encounter difficulties can be taught certain skills in a lighthearted manner. You can develop their self-confidence by leading them in exercises that they will be able to do without difficulty. Once they have gained self-confidence, they will have no problem with the more difficult exercises.

Of course, a child's age in years does not tell you everything. Some 6-year-olds may have an experiential age of 4, and vice versa. When putting a group together, focus on matching their levels of experience and social and motor skills. Whether they have racked up the same exact number of years is less important. With that caveat, here are the age groups we recommend:

Preschoolers: 3–5 Years Old

Preschoolers are busy learning how to use space and having fun with all the different ways they can move around. They discover space through play, and delight in discovering their physical potential. They learn how to hop, stand on one leg, wink, run, walk backwards, hobble, make silly gestures—you name it. Yoga for this age group should involve total-body movements—movements that involve the whole body, are easily explained and understood, are often spontaneous, and don't involve complicated details. Avoid correcting preschoolers when they are doing yoga.

At this age children have wonderful powers of fantasy, as you can see in the games they play together. We can use these powers of fantasy in the yoga games. Joining in children's enthusiasm, taking part in their fantasies and games, stimulating their discoveries, and understanding their delight are the leader's happy responsibilities. Preschoolers move easily and their efforts quickly tire them out. On the other hand, they also recover their energy quickly. Keep exercises short and lively to help the children maintain their energy and concentration. Young children love repetition: If you use a certain opening or goodbye song for one class session, they may delight in hearing it at every single class thereafter. Preschoolers identify primarily with their parents or other caretakers. They are often cautious about playing with others. You can help them discover that cooperation can be fun by occasionally asking them to hold hands and work together on a simple exercise.

Children are eager to learn at this age, but they are also easily distracted; time means little to them. This can cause frustration for the leader, as lessons don't last forever and you may want to achieve certain goals. Telling young children your plans in advance and repeatedly may help them move from one thing to the next in a timely fashion.

A final and important note: At this age children have a very soft bone structure and lots of cartilage. Hanging positions stretch these structures, and jumps can quickly overtax them. Be very careful with this type of exercise!

Elementary School Children in Kindergarten Through Second Grade: 5–8 Years Old

By this time children are becoming stronger and gaining more control over their movements. The delicate motor system is starting to develop. They are physically almost tireless and learn more and more easily. They begin to develop the desire for variation. For the leader this means, for example, no longer rounding off with the same song each week.

By this time children are using fantasy games to explore their emotions and play with different role models. The difference between fantasy and reality is not always clear for children of this age group. The imaginary witch can become so vivid that for the children it becomes a frightening reality. As leader, always take this into account.

Every day the children are growing in strength, dexterity, and independence. Because they are able to do more and more, it can be hard for children to know when to stop. As leader, you must help them find their boundaries. Make sure they do not over-stretch, over-tire, or otherwise harm themselves. Children trust their caretakers and their own environment implicitly and are unaware of the dangers. It is up to you to keep them safe.

Important friendships begin to be formed at this point. Children are learning to cooperate and take more of an interest in each other. Encourage this by having them work together in pairs and groups more often. Abstract concepts, such as freedom, security, loss, and generosity, begin to take on meaning. You can use the games in the section "Lessons with a Theme" to explore these concepts through movement.

Elementary School Children in Third Through Fifth Grade: 8–11 Years Old

In this phase we see the fantasy world begin to fade and the interest in reality increase. Children don't want to pretend to be a baker any more; they want to help bake real bread. Home is still a safe haven, but outside is "real life," and the child enjoys more and more activities outside the home. In yoga class, children of this age love change, are more businesslike, and want fewer fantasy exercises.

This is the best age to learn good technique. The children become very dexterous, often more so than adults. By now children can perform a wide variety of movements. They love to move; fast equals fun. Children this age often love to perform and be the best at something. It is up to the leader to take advantage of the children's drive and agility, give them direction, inspire them, but also to slow them down when necessary (for instance, where there are risks the children cannot foresee). Help them remember that yoga is not a competitive sport: Rather, it is about the joy of movement and self-improvement, not competing to stretch the farthest and fastest. Children who strive to outdo each other risk injuring themselves.

Friendships become very important. Toward the end of this stage, the child wants to stand out from the others but be part of a group at the same time. Boys ride their bikes at breakneck speed. Girls begin to feel like women. Since children assimilate a lot of information from the media and their peers and teachers, they may develop opinions that surprise their parents. They are beginning the long process of transformation from children to adults.

Yoga in the Classroom

Yoga does not have to be confined to the studio or gym. Many yoga exercises are perfectly suited to an ordinary classroom. Some exercises need a little adaptation—such as sitting on a chair with your feet on the ground instead of sitting or lying on the floor. Others can be done while standing next to a desk.

When children are very rowdy or listless, they can be calmed down or brightened up with breathing exercises. These exercises have a harmonizing effect. Trust and cooperation exercises have a positive influence on their behavior toward each other. These games teach children mutual respect.

If you make yoga a part of your classroom routine, you will find it doesn't interfere with your lesson plan. On the contrary, the children perform better. There is less fear of failure, so they have more self-confidence. This stimulates academic performance.

Information for the Leader: A Positive Approach

When we see children running, full of enthusiasm, to yoga class, our primary goal is to maintain that level of joy. Teaching and guiding children entails finding a balance between the things you want to teach them and the various things they want to do. How can you approach each lesson in the most positive way? By allowing space for children's creativity within the possibilities of the lesson.

Planning a Yoga Session: How to Combine Games

Each of the yoga games can stand alone. You can also combine several games to form an hour-long yoga session. The games are grouped according to type, and each section begins with a brief introduction about the type of game covered. You can put your own lessons together by, for instance, choosing one game or exercise from each subject. The following types of game are included:

- breathing exercises and games

- yoga postures and movements

- relaxation

- sitting still: a meditative exercise

- cooperation and trust games

The final section, "Lessons with a Theme," shows how an hour-long yoga session can be built up. This section includes several lessons based on lighthearted themes such as the seasons, celebrations, and animals, as well as serious subjects such as loss. Each lesson has an introduction, and each involves breathing exercises, poses, movement, cooperation, and relaxation. Effort and rest should alternate. Always give children the opportunity to share their experiences of the exercises and to talk about them.

Workspace

Yoga does not require any particular type of space. You can do it almost anywhere. Still, certain spaces work better for young children than others. Children are spontaneous and lively and need space to be themselves. They want to run around, jump up and down, and make noise, so make sure your workspace is big enough. If mats will not be provided, have children bring in a mat, towel, or blanket to sit on. This will help each child create a space for herself in the room. Children also need space in a figurative sense, so let them bring in their own ideas and creativity. You will find that you can learn a lot from them. Give yourself space as well: Use your own enthusiasm, imagination, and creativity to make something special out of the lesson.

You may want to have certain props on hand so that you can try out good, spontaneous ideas—things like tennis balls, ping-pong balls, cotton balls, straws, balloons, cloths, rope, and sticks. Cushions are good for sitting on, and a good sound system will be needed as well, since many of the games involve music. Of course the floor should be clean, as many of the games involve lying on the floor. The temperature should be comfortable and it should be possible to open a window during the breathing exercises so that everyone can feel and smell the fresh air.

The Leader's Role

The leader plays many important roles in conducting these yoga games: guide, cheerleader, moderator, coach, spotter, and more. Here are a few tips for leading the games. As leader, be sure to do the following:

- **Present the exercises and games to the children in a warm, open manner without any sort of pressure.** Try to be sensitive to the reasons why children might be overexcited or sluggish and ask them how they are feeling. Be flexible and ready to change the structure of the lesson to their needs, even if you had other plans in mind.

- **Give children positive attention.** Help them understand that everyone has different strengths and talents. Emphasize the noncompetitive nature of the yoga games: Children should focus on enjoying the exercises and doing what feels right; they should not compete to be the best or laugh at others who have difficulty with certain exercises. Everyone can work in his own way.

- **Be clear about how you want children to behave in class.** Children like a direct approach. Tell them if there is something happening that you don't like and explain why. Talk to them in a way suited to their age. Encourage the children to monitor their own behavior, as well. Yoga will help them develop their own inner discipline.

- **Create a good atmosphere to begin the lesson.** If you are teaching yoga to children who are coming after school, you can begin by giving them a drink of water or juice. The children will calm down and can talk about what happened in school today or since the last yoga class. (If you are working with preschool children, the lessons will be shorter and having a drink first may take too much of your time. Start right in with relaxation exercises.)

- **Respect children's ideas.** Often, children come up with terrific ideas. Being flexible enough to try out children's ideas can make your class much more interesting. Just as often, though, children want (or think they want) to do the same things over and over. The children come in full of expectation: "Are we going to play mirrors today?" "Are we going to do the salutation to the sun today?" In that situation you might say: "This time I've got something special for you, so we need the whole hour. Remind me to play the mirror game again next week. If you like, you can practice at home in the meantime and show it to us next week." Acknowledge children's ideas, and accommodate them if you can, but give them the benefits of your own ideas and leadership.

- **Help the children in a group get to know each other.** You might begin every class by having all the children sit in a circle and call out their names. This can be done in all kinds of fun ways. Each child in turn can make up her own movement to go with her name. Older children could make up a movement for each syllable. You could greet each child by name yourself, or challenge one of the children to do the same. Alternatively, each child could call out the name of the child to his left. You can turn the name game into a story: "I'm Nicky and I'm going on a journey." As you go around the circle, each child adds the names of the children who went before him: "I'm Marco and I'm going on a journey. I'm taking Nicky with me." "I'm Alisha and I'm going on a journey. I'm taking Marco and Nicky with me." Make sure the children learn each other's names. When they know each other's names, children become more conscious and considerate of each other. It is the start of learning how to be sociable.

- **Watch out for hazards such as candy and jewelry.** Now and then, a child might bring candies or chewing gum to the class. Explain that it is dangerous to do yoga while eating and offer to keep the gum or candy safe until after class is over. Jewelry is another common danger. Point out what could go wrong: "If you're leaning on your hands, that bracelet may get caught underneath and hurt you. See what I mean? So take the jewelry off before we start. I know you really love this bracelet so I'll keep it for you and we'll be sure it doesn't get broken."

- **Ask the children to use the bathroom before class begins.** "Can I go to the bathroom?" asks Suzie in the middle of the lesson. And suddenly everyone wants to go. To prevent this from becoming a habit, it's a good idea to ask the children to go before the class starts. It is such a pity to interrupt the atmosphere to let children go out. When they change clothes before class they can go to the bathroom and wash their hands.

- **Encourage friends to find their independence.** Some of the games are for pairs, and you may find that certain couples always want to work together. Keeping the same partner is limiting because the children never get the chance to discover different people's ideas and styles. You can discourage this by forming couples arbitrarily: You might have the children count off, or simply assign partners yourself. Some friends may still insist on working together. Breaking this habit and keeping everyone happy requires some organizational genius on the part of the leader. For example, perhaps Malik always works with Justin and Brandon always works with Jessica. For a mirroring exercise, you might suggest: "Why don't you work as a foursome? Jessica, you stand next to Brandon, because you're friends. Malik and Justin stand facing them. Jessica, you be Malik's mirror, and Brandon, you be Justin's mirror." This solution lets the couples stay together but still do the exercise with someone else.

  Some couples stay together even when everyone else is moving independently. In some cases, this can hamper their creativity. If this becomes a habit, point it out to the children involved without making judgements or putting pressure on them. They may decide to try working independently.

- **Help children to laugh with each other, not at each other.** Some days, children just feel giggly—anything can inspire a fit of giggles. If children are laughing at each other's mistakes, clothes, and so on, this can be very hurtful. Instead of using giggling to exclude, help children make giggling into a fun game in which everyone is included. For instance, perhaps a child wears shocking pink leggings to class and everyone starts to laugh. You might say: "Hey, it's nice to hear how happy her leggings make you! Have you seen my silly new

T-shirt?" After everyone giggles at the T-shirt, give each child a turn to find something to laugh about. Then say: "Giggling is great when we all do it together. Keep an eye on that so people don't misunderstand you. It's not nice if people think you're making fun of them. We can all laugh together!"

- **Teach the children to pay attention to you and to each other.** Some of the games call for children to perform for the group—perhaps to show each other a movement they have thought up. Encourage the group to be supportive when others are performing. Explain that it is exciting and, for some children, just a bit scary to be out in front alone. Tell them: "Watch carefully and remember that when it's your turn you will want everyone to pay attention. Smile at each other. That helps people show their ideas without being shy."

- **Make sure children understand when an exercise requires quiet.** You might introduce the relaxation exercises by saying, "In the next few minutes try to be very quiet so that you can feel and see inside yourself." If someone starts talking enthusiastically during a silent exercise, remind him to be quiet for now, and as soon as the exercise is over, invite him to share his idea.

- **Make use of children's energy; don't try to squelch them.** It goes without saying that as a teacher you need a huge amount of flexibility. This means that you can plan your lessons in principle, but still leave lots of space for the children. Sometimes a group will be very talkative, giggly, and fidgety. You may find that the lesson you planned just won't work. Instead, concentrate on the children and their unusual amount of energy. You might let them move freely for a while, and then have each child think up a movement for the class to imitate. Keep the focus positive, and try to make them aware of their own energy: "Today is special because you've all got so much energy. Sometimes your body is so full of energy that you've just got to keep going. Everyone has thought up a movement. I've enjoyed being with you today. See you next week." No matter what their energy level, the children are always welcome and there is room for all their movement.

Key to the Icons Used in the Games

To help you find games suitable for a particular situation, all the games are coded with symbols or icons. These icons tell you at a glance some things about the game:

- the appropriate grade level/age group
- the amount of time needed
- the organization of the players
- the props required
- the space required

These are explained in more detail below.

Suitability in terms of age The games are designed for children ages 3 through 11. The recommended age groups correspond to grade level divisions commonly used in the educational system:

 = Children in preschool through grade 5 (ages 3 through 11)

 = Young children in kindergarten through grade 2 (ages 5 through 8)

= Older children in grades 3 through 5 (ages 8 through 11)

How long the game takes The games are divided into those that require about 5 minutes or less, 10 minutes, 15 minutes, 20 minutes, and those that require 1 hour.

5 minutes or less   10 minutes   15 minutes

20 minutes   1 hour

The organization of players All of the games can be adapted to virtually any size of group. The grouping icons indicate how players will be organized to play the game: in pairs, in small groups, or all together as a group.

 = Players will work in pairs.

 = Players will work in small groups.

 = All the players will work together as a group.

Amount of space needed The games that require an especially large amount of space, such as a gymnasium, are marked with the following icon:

 = Large space needed

Whether you need props Most of the games require no special props. In some cases, art materials, blindfolds, natural objects, or other simple props will enhance the game. These games are flagged with the following icon, and the necessary materials are listed next to the Props heading:

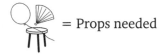 = Props needed

Breathing Exercises and Games

This section contains short exercises and games to help the children become more aware of their breathing. The breath is the mirror of how we feel. Through conscious breathing we can change our tension into relaxation.

How Breathing Works

The diaphragm is tireless—it keeps us breathing 24 hours a day. This domed muscle divides the chest cavity from the abdominal cavity and lies like a blanket over our organs. When the diaphragm is tensed, it pushes the organs of the belly downwards and increases the size of the chest cavity. This causes a change in pressure that forces the lungs to expand and suck in air. The expanding lungs and shifting organs cause the whole torso to expand, moving outward at the chest, belly, sides, and back. When the diaphragm relaxes, the size of the chest cavity decreases, the lungs expel air, and the torso shrinks inward. This is a normal breathing movement that happens no matter what position a person is in.

During active exercise, the intercostal muscles (the muscles between the ribs) assist the diaphragm to produce deeper breathing. The lower ribs spread apart and expand the chest cavity further. More air comes into the lungs, providing oxygen for dynamic movements. This extra lung capacity is also useful in singing.

The Four Stages of Breathing

If we watch the breathing process, we see four stages: inhalation, rest (with lungs full), exhalation, and rest (with lungs empty). The inhalation represents the feeling of "self," receiving, and making a place for yourself on the earth. As we breathe in, we draw power into ourselves. The rest with lungs full represents strength. Exhalation represents the feeling of "other," giving, and letting go—but also powerful expression as in screaming. The rest with empty lungs represents silence and trust—in your own body and in everything.

In the Classroom

Children often become fidgety in class. Beginning a class with breathing exercises can have a calming effect. The children reflect on themselves, and this makes them quieter and better able to concentrate. Breathing exercises can also be helpful before classroom presentations. When children become nervous about speaking in front of the class, they may unconsciously tense their face and neck muscles, constricting their airway and making speaking difficult. Deep breathing can help them relax.

Game 1 (Breathing with Awareness) and game 2 (Belly Breathing) are very effective in the classroom. For these exercises it is possible for the children to sit on their chairs instead of lying down as indicated. They can place their feet firmly on the ground and put their hands on their bellies. You can adapt almost all the exercises and games for the classroom in this manner. If the weather allows, open the windows during breathing exercises so the children can feel the fresh air.

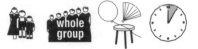

Breathing with Awareness

Props: mats (optional)

Breathing is something we do automatically, without thinking. We can control the breath and use it consciously, however. Feeling and observing the movement of the breath is the first and most important step.

Have the children lie down on a mat in whatever position they find comfortable. Encourage them to lie as still as possible. Then ask: "Are any parts of your body still moving? Where is your body moving inside?"

Children lying on their backs may notice their chests or bellies rising and falling with each breath. If children lie on their bellies, their lower backs and bottoms may rise and fall with the breath. Go around the room to each child. Put your hand gently on the part of each child's body that is rising and falling with the breath. Say: "That's nice. Can you feel that it's moving here?"

Explain that each time we breathe in, we take air into our lungs. The lungs fill with air and get bigger, just like a balloon. When we breathe out, the air empties out of our lungs and they get smaller again. We can see and feel our lungs getting bigger and smaller with each breath, because they move the chest, belly, or back up and down.

Variations:

- If this exercise is undertaken just after the children have finished exercising, they may feel the breath higher up in the chest. They may be able to feel the heartbeat as well.

- Have children lie in different positions, rolling onto their backs, bellies, or sides. Ask what parts of their bodies are moving now.

- Have children do this exercise while sitting or standing. The breathing movements will be more subtle, so children will have to concentrate.

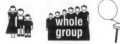

Belly Breathing

Props: mats (optional)

We breathe automatically, but not all of us breathe well or efficiently. Many people develop bad breathing habits, such as chest breathing. (See the introduction to this section on pages 14–15.) We can use conscious breathing to direct the breath downward, into the belly instead of the chest. When the breath makes the belly expand, that shows we are using the diaphragm muscle to fill the lungs entirely.

Lead the children through game 1 (Breathing with Awareness). Then have them lie on their backs and place their hands on their bellies. Ask whether their bellies rise and fall as they breathe. Encourage the children to guide the breath into their bellies. When they inhale, the belly should grow bigger, like a balloon. When they exhale, the belly should shrink. Tell the children they should not force the movement: They should let the lungs lift their bellies from the inside.

Afterward, ask the children how it felt to breathe into their bellies.

Variation: People often tend to use chest breathing when they exercise. Have the group do some aerobic exercise until they are breathing hard, and then do the belly breathing exercise. It will be harder to control the breath, but the change from chest to belly breathing will be more dramatic.

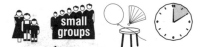

Airball

Props: a plastic drinking straw for each player and a cotton ball (or crumpled ball of paper) for each team

In this breathing game, players use straws to blow cotton balls around. Breathing through a straw encourages players to inhale and exhale more deeply. They learn to use their diaphragms and abdominal muscles to control the exhalation.

   Give a straw to each child and have teams of about five players lie on their bellies in a circle. Place a cotton ball in front of one of the team members and tell players they must pass it all the way around the circle, so that every player has a turn. There is one catch: Players cannot touch the ball with their hands, straws, or anything else! If the players have difficulty figuring out how to put the straws to use, explain that players can move the ball by blowing on it through the straws.

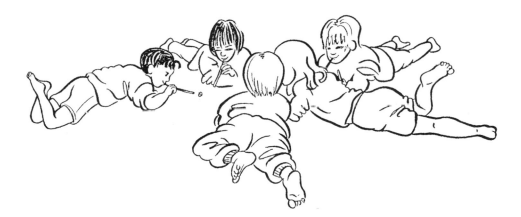

After teams are finished, ask them how it felt to breathe through a straw.

Variations:

- Have each team sit around a table instead of lying on the ground.

- Instead of blowing on the ball, have players pick it up by sucking it onto the end of the straw. Each player should pick up the ball, place it in front of the next child, and let it go. This variation focuses on the inhalation rather than on the exhalation.

Air
Soccer

Props: a plastic drinking straw for each player, a ping-pong ball for each soccer match, small boxes to use as goals

Like game 3 (Airball), this game trains the exhalation. Pass out straws to everybody and divide the group into teams of three to five players. You will need two teams of equal number for each soccer match. (For example, a class of 28 could have two matches with five-player teams and a third match with four-player teams.) Have each team choose a member to be the goalie.

Players can lie on their bellies or sit around a table. The two goalies should be at either end of the "playing field" with the goals in front of them. (To make the goals, you might tape small cardboard boxes—e.g. shoeboxes—on their sides so that the open tops face out.) The other players line up alternately on the sides (see illustration). Start the ping-pong ball in the center of the playing field and begin play. The object is to blow the ball into the opposing team's goal, without ever touching the ball.

You can play to a time limit or up to the first three goals.

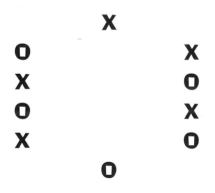

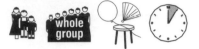

Blowing Leaves

Props: a leaf for each player

In a playful manner, this game teaches children how to control the breath, blowing alternately hard and soft. Seat the group in a circle and hand out leaves. Have children place the leaves in their open palms and blow gently on the leaves. Say: "Notice what happens in your body when you blow."

Next, have the children blow hard on the leaves, like a gusty storm. Ask how this feels different. Invite children to experiment with different ways of blowing on the leaves. Afterward, have them discuss what happens to the leaves and what happens inside as they blow in different ways.

See game 57 on page 108 (Fall) for ideas on how to incorporate these activities into an hour-long yoga lesson.

Variations:

- Have children stand in a circle, throw their leaves into the air, and blow them towards the center of the circle.

- Have children lie on their bellies with one cheek on the ground. Place a leaf just in front of each child's face and challenge the children to blow the leaves into the air.

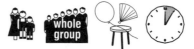

Seeing the Breath

Props: a cotton ball for each child

This exercise helps the children get to know their breathing patterns.

Seat the children in a circle and give each one a cotton ball. Have them place the cotton balls on their open palms and then hold them right under their noses. Ask them to watch the balls carefully. Then ask:

What do you see? Try to breathe normally, through your nose. Can you tell from the movement of the cotton whether you are breathing in, pausing the breath with lungs full, breathing out, or pausing with empty lungs?

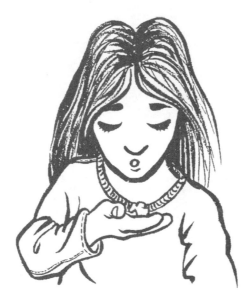

Variations:

- Have children breathe through the mouth.

- Invite them to yawn.

- Try the activity when children are breathing heavily from aerobic exercise.

See game 60 on page 117 (Snow) and game 61 on page 121 (The Balloon's Journey) for ideas on how to incorporate this activity into an hour-long themed lesson.

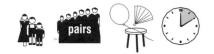

Air
Volley

Props: a ping-pong ball for each pair of players; cardboard scraps, toilet paper tubes, or small boxes (optional)

Have players lie on the ground in pairs, or sit opposite each other at a table. Give each pair a ping-pong ball and ask partners to pass their ball back and forth without touching it. Partners can gently blow on the ball to make it move. Challenge pairs to keep the ball going back and forth as long as they can without letting it fall off the table or roll out of reach.

Variations:

- Have partners blow the ball back and forth through a tunnel. You might make the tunnel out of cardboard scraps or a cardboard toilet paper tube.

- Make two goals out of small cardboard boxes or cardboard scraps. Players can try to blow the ball into their partner's goal, while defending their own goal.

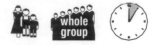

Feeling the Breath

This exercise helps children become familiar with their own breathing patterns.

Seat the children in a circle. Ask them to hold one hand loosely in front of the nose and mouth. Tell the group: "Close your eyes and think about your hand. Can you feel when you breathe in, pause, breathe out, and pause again?"

Invite players to experiment with different ways of breathing. Players could breathe through their mouths or noses, yawn, and breathe as hard and as lightly as they can. Ask them if they can make their breath feel cool (by blowing through pursed lips, as if cooling soup) and hot (by opening the mouth and breathing "hah," as if warming hands).

After a few minutes, ask players what they could feel.

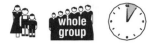

Opening the Throat

Many people constrict their throats when they are feeling nervous, upset, or excited. A closed throat can make exercising, using the voice, and even breathing difficult. This exercise helps players recognize what a relaxed, open throat feels like.

Have the group sit in a circle and help them loosen their neck and shoulder muscles with a few warm-ups. You might have them tense their shoulders, raising them up to their ears, and then relax them. Now ask the children to yawn. Encourage them to notice how their throats feel when they yawn. Tell them that this is the feeling of an open throat.

Next, ask children to sit up as tall as possible. They should imagine someone pulling up on the crown of their heads with a string. Have them say "hah" softly with an open throat. As children vocalize, have them drop their heads down to their chests, and then bring them back up. Then have children drop their heads backwards and to each side, bringing the head back to center each time. Ask them how the positions feel different. Help them recognize that bending the neck constricts the throat, and that the throat is most open in the center position. Point out how standing straight can help with breathing freely.

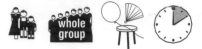

Breath on the Window

Props: clear glass windows within children's reach

This game is best suited for a damp day in winter, when breath mist lingers longer on the glass.

Invite the children to stand by the windows. Point out that it's possible to make your breath hot or cold: Blowing through pursed lips cools soup, while breathing "hah" with open mouth warms hands. Show the children how they can breathe a mist onto the glass with open mouth and throat. Now they can make a quick drawing on the window. If the images last long enough, each child can show her drawing, tell what it is, and discuss why she chose to draw that picture.

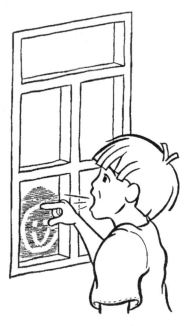

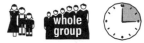

Sounds

This exercise helps children understand how their bodies produce sound. They can feel different parts of their heads, throats, chests, and so on vibrating as they concentrate on creating different sounds. They learn to feel where in the body the power behind each sound originates. They think about how the mouth, lungs, and throat work to create sound. In addition, the exercise helps train children's abdominal muscles and increase their breath capacity.

Have the children sit in a circle. Invite them to yawn and feel that wonderful open sensation in their throats. Tell them they are going to make some sounds, and ask them to keep their throats as open and relaxed as they can. Then lead them in making a series of sounds:

Breathe slowly, deep into your belly. We are going to make a long mmmmm sound. /m/ is a nice sound because you can feel your lips buzzing together and itching! We call that "vibrating."

Make the sound yourself so that people are not shy. The sound can be made on different notes. This usually sounds very nice when everyone does it together. You might choose a number of the sounds below to explore and discuss with children:

- *What parts of your face vibrate when you make the /m/ sound? The /n/ sound? The /r/ sound? The /th/ sound in "the"? The /v/ sound? The /z/ sound?*

- *How do you move your lips and tongue to make the /b/ sound? The /d/ sound? The /f/ sound? The /l/ sound? The /p/ sound? The /t/ sound? The /th/ sound in "thin"? The /s/ sound? The /w/ sound?*

- *What happens inside your mouth when you make the /ch/ sound? The hard /g/ sound (as in "get")? The /h/ sound? The /k/ sound? The /j/ sound? The /sh/ sound? The /y/ sound?*

- *Which vowel sound makes your mouth feel more open, /ee/ or /ah/? (/ah/) Which of these feels more open, /oh/ or /oo/? (/oh/) (Other open vowels are /eh/ and /uh/; short /a/ [as in "cat"] is a closed vowel.) Where can you feel the different vowel sounds vibrating as you make them?*

Variations:

- Have the children do these exercises while standing or walking.

- Invite the children to cover their ears while they make the sounds, to help them concentrate on the vibrations inside their heads.

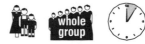

Singing Names

This is a very nice way for children to learn each other's names. When you pronounce a child's name clearly and slowly, with much care and attention, you serenade him. The child will grow before your eyes.

Seat the group in a circle. Explain that you are going to go around the circle and sing each player's name, and you would like everyone to join in. Breathe in before beginning a name, and sing each one on a long out-breath. Take each name and draw out all the sounds you can, chanting them as slowly and clearly as you can.

"What sound does Angela's name begin with? Yes, with *Aaaa*. Do you want to join in? *Aaannngeeelllaaa*."

Note: Of course, some consonant sounds (/b/, /k/, /d/, /g/, /j/, /p/, /t/) cannot be drawn out. Simply focus on the sounds that you can linger over.

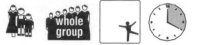

Animal Sounds

As every child knows, animals all have their own distinct sounds. A bee buzzes, a lion roars, a crow caws, a snake hisses, a frog croaks, and so on.

This game helps stimulate children's imagination and spontaneity. Because the children move freely around the room as they make the noises, they also learn about the use of physical space. They learn to express themselves both through the voice and through the body.

Choose an animal and invite the group to think up all the sounds it makes. Children can move around the room, imitating the motions of that animal as they recreate its sounds. You might use the examples below.

Bird: Help young children practice whistling. Tell them: "Tighten your mouth into a small circle. Put one hand on your belly so you can feel it going in and out. Hold the other hand a few inches in front of your mouth and see if you can feel the air as you blow it out. Now see if you can make a sound. First very quietly...and now louder."

Bee: Invite children to pretend they are bees visiting all the colorful flowers in a garden. Encourage them to make the buzzing sound of a bee. Have the children stand still and hold their hands over their ears as they buzz. How does this change the feel of the sound?

Lion: Ask children to imagine they are big, powerful lions. Tell them: "Walk on your hands and feet around the room. Imagine that you are a big strong lion. Let everyone hear how strong you are!"

Afterward, have the group discuss what it was like to make the sounds of the different animals. How did the sounds make them feel?

Variation: Let the children choose their own animals and sounds.

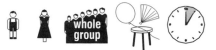

Side Breathing

Props: mats

Most of us don't fill our lungs to capacity. Filling the unused space in the lungs can greatly increase our endurance. Practicing side breathing and belly breathing (see game 2 on page 18) will help children fill their lungs and avoid shallow chest breathing. Side breathing also gives the ribs and spine more mobility and prevents stiffness.

Have children lie on their sides with the top hand on the lower ribs. Tell them: "Breathe in deeply and feel your ribs spreading apart. Notice how your hand rises with the breath. Keep your breathing slow and relaxed, and remember to breathe out all the way."

After a couple of minutes, have children roll onto the other side and repeat the exercise.

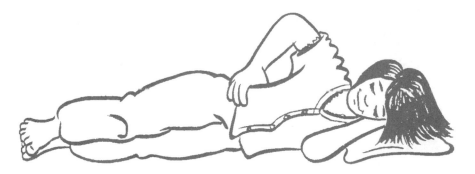

Variation: Instead of lying down, have children sit to do this exercise. As they breathe in, ask children to raise one arm like a wing, above their heads. The arm movement should be slow and sweeping, like the wing of a big seagull. Encourage children to move the ribs outwards as much as they can, by directing the breath to their side. On the exhale they bring the arm down again. After doing this about six times, have children switch to the other arm.

Note: The movement and the breath should both be slow and relaxed. With side breathing, the breath is much deeper and the lungs take in much more air. If you don't keep this exercise slow, the children may hyperventilate, becoming dizzy or light-headed.

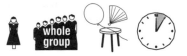

Back Breathing

Props: a wall with enough clear space for all the children to sit against it

This exercise is difficult, because the back is a part of the body we don't think about very often.

Have children sit with their backs against the wall. Ask them to close their eyes and become aware of the wall. Tell them:

Feel the support of the floor and the wall. Think about what parts of your back are touching the wall. Imagine your back is covered with ink, and you are stamping a mark on the wall. What shape is the mark? The next time you inhale, try to send the air into your back. Feel how your back becomes wider and makes more contact with the wall. In the lower part of the back especially, you can feel your back pressing against the wall as you breathe in and moving away as you breathe out again.

Variations:

- Have children lie on the ground and feel how the contact with the ground changes. As above, guide them to send their breath to the back.

- Have children work in pairs. One child lies on his belly and the other child kneels next to him and puts her hands on his back. The hands of the kneeling child move as the child who is lying down breathes in and out.

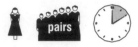

Feeling Sounds Through the Back

Divide the group into pairs. Have partners sit back to back, either on chairs (with the back of the chair turned to the side) or on the ground. Encourage players to think about how their backs feel when they sit this way.

Now ask one partner to make a sound—perhaps singing, or talking, or just saying "hah." Ask the other partner where in her back she felt the sound, and what it felt like. Now let the other partner make a sound. Invite partners to experiment with making various sounds. How do the sounds feel different? Can they all be felt in the same area, or do they resonate in different places?

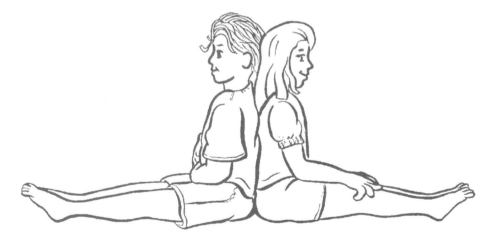

Yoga Postures and Movements

This section contains a number of adaptations of more traditional yoga postures and movements. Along with the description of each posture is an explanation of its benefits.

A child in his natural state is a child in movement. As he moves, he playfully strikes spontaneous poses—reaching into the air, curled into a ball, crouched like a crab, whatever his body feels like at that moment. Many of these positions can be found amongst the yoga *asanas*. These are specific postures that have harmonizing and energizing effects. Just as a good walk through the woods can be relaxing for an overactive child and activity peps up a quiet child, these *asanas* help to bring about balance.

Watch the children to make sure that they don't hold their breath in order to achieve or hold a certain posture. Encourage them to breathe in and out gently and in a steady rhythm. If the children become too focused on imitating poses perfectly, they may force their bodies into place. They can never create harmony this way, and they run the risk of injuring themselves. As soon as the idea of performance comes in, we lose the notion of yoga. The most important thing is pleasure in movement.

A full discussion of the *asanas* lies beyond the scope of this book. There are some *asanas* we actively discourage for children: headstand *(sirasana)*, full candle pose, fish pose *(matsyasana)*, hero pose *(virasana)*, warrior pose *(virabhadrasana)*, and the half body twist *(ardha matsyendrasana)*. A child's body is quite fragile. The bone structure is still soft, and cartilage and connective tissues are easily damaged. The fact that many exercises are easy for the children to learn does not mean that these exercises are good for their young bodies.

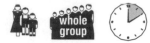

The
Mountain

One of the things we do in yoga is develop awareness of how we stand. Standing firmly means that we feel strong. From a balanced stance we can move the body in powerful ways. This is why the base on which you stand is so important. We stand in bare feet so that we can feel the ground and make contact with the earth. Bare feet are the best shoes for yoga.

Have the children stand in a line side by side, spaced a foot or so apart. You might instruct them as follows:

Feel your feet touching the ground. Stamp your feet a few times, then stop. What parts of your feet are pressing into the ground? Do you have more weight on your toes, or on your heels? Try to spread your weight out evenly across your whole foot. If you are standing on the inside part of your foot, try to shift your weight more to the outside of your feet in order to create an even distribution of weight. Make sure each foot is carrying the same amount of weight. Feel yourself firmly rooted to the ground.

Now think about your legs. How do your calves, knees, and thighs feel? Make sure your knees are not locked in place: Shake them out a little and leave them just slightly bent. Stand tall, with a straight back. Let your arms hang down straight at your sides. Make sure your shoulders are not rising up toward your ears: Keep the shoulders loose, not tense. Hold your head high and straight, with your chin tucked in a little. Imagine someone is pulling up the top of your head with a string. You are a tall, steady mountain.

Invite the group to sing a song as they stand, to the tune of a drill sergeant's chant:

call: I'm a mountain straight and tall

response: I'm a mountain straight and tall

call: The strongest wind can't make me fall

response: The strongest wind can't make me fall

call: Forward, back

response: Forward, back

call: Left, right

response: Left, right

together: Forward, back, left, right, forward, back, LEFT, RIGHT!

As children sing "forward, back, left, right," they should hold hands and rock their bodies in the direction the song says. Ask them to keep their feet rooted in place. (In other words, when children sing "forward," they should rock forward on their toes. When they sing "back," they should rock back on their heels, and so on.)

Variations:

- Instead of merely rocking to the left and right, have players shift their weight completely and stand first on the left leg, then on the right leg.

- Have players stand on their toes as they sing and move to the song.

- Have players stand on their heels as they sing and move to the song.

- Instead of having children sing the song, simply ask them to rock forward on their toes, then back on their heels, and then side to side. This way they can do the movement more consciously.

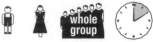

The
Tree

This pose helps children develop their strength and balance. Good physical balance has a positive effect on mental and emotional balance.

The traditional tree position is a stance on one foot with the hands together above the head (see illustration on page 41). Demonstrate this posture first and then help the children ease into it step by step. Have children spread out around the room and begin in the mountain pose (see game 17 on page 38). You might instruct them as follows:

Stand tall and feel the ground under your feet. Without lifting your feet, transfer your weight to one foot, then to the other foot. Choose one foot and put all your weight on it. Concentrate on how it feels to stand with your weight on this foot alone. Wait until you feel steady. Then, keeping your weight on one foot, gently move the other foot. You can brush your foot along the ground. Once you can do this easily, lift the foot slightly off the ground. Concentrate on the weight keeping you steady on the ground. The leg you are standing on is what is keeping you upright. The other leg is hanging free. Now bend your free leg and put your foot as high as you can on the inner part of the leg you are standing on. If you need to, put your arms out to help you balance.

When you feel steady, slowly raise your arms above your head. If you can, put your palms together. Remember to keep breathing gently in and out. Feel how strong you are in this position. Feel your hands pointing up to the sky and your feet firmly planted on the earth. When you are ready, you can bring your foot down and stand on both feet again.

Have children switch feet and repeat the exercise. Then discuss it together.

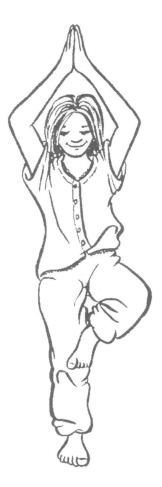

Variation: If children have difficulty balancing, you might have them steady themselves by touching a wall with one hand. When they gain confidence, they can lift their hands from the wall and balance without aid.

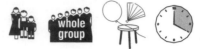

Sitting Postures

Props: mats

By about 9 months, most babies sit up beautifully straight without any support. Sitting up straight is easy for young children, but it becomes difficult as we grow older. Lounging on sofas and bending over desks, we learn to slouch. Many of these yoga games involve sitting, so use this exercise to make sure the children understand how to sit in a well-grounded position, with a straight spine.

Have the group stand in a circle. Invite them to think of lots of different ways to sit on the ground. Ask a volunteer to show the group a way to sit on the floor with a straight back. Have everyone follow her example. Then instruct the children as follows:

Feel the ground underneath you. Does it feel solid? Is it hard or soft? Now imagine you have roots going down from your body, like a

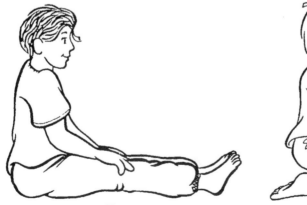

staff pose

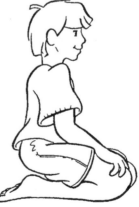

kneeling pose

plant, and send your roots into the ground. Are you sitting more firmly now?

Now lean forward. Can you feel more pressure in front as you do this? Now lean back—do you feel more pressure behind you as you do that? Now move to one side. Does that also put more pressure on the ground? Now lean to the other side. Can you feel more pressure there also? Next we are going to lean forward, to the side, back, and to the other side, going around in a circle. Stay on the ground; don't lift your legs or buttocks. Feel the pressure on the different parts of your body as you go around in a circle. Now turn a circle in the other direction.

Make the circle smaller and smaller until you come to a stop. How does it feel to sit still? Are you sitting differently now?

Now that the children are grounded in this particular sitting position, have them do an activity in the position. You might choose from the list of sitting activities below. Afterward, invite a new volunteer to demonstrate a different sitting position and repeat the exercise above. Make sure all the basic yoga sitting positions are covered (see illustration). You can do a different activity in each position.

Sitting Activities:
- move the shoulders in circles forward and backward, first together and then one by one

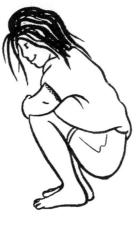

squat

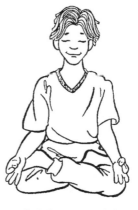

full lotus position

- keeping the back straight, drop the head forward and slowly bring it back upright

- turn the head from left to right

- raise both arms above the head and back down again, like a bird stretching its wings

- first raise one arm, then the other

- raise both arms and make yourself as tall as you can

- make funny faces

- make funny sounds (see games 11–13 on pages 29–32)

Note: Children may sit in a half-lotus or a simple cross-legged position if the lotus position is too difficult. Tell them not to force their bodies into a pose that feels uncomfortable. In the half-lotus position, the legs are crossed and one foot is placed on top of the opposite thigh, while the other foot rests on the floor.

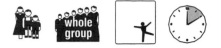

The **Frog**

♪ **Music:** background music (optional)

Squatting helps keep the legs limber. By hopping like frogs, children strengthen their muscles through play.

Have the children squat, bending their knees out to the sides and lowering their bottoms almost to the floor. Encourage them to try putting their palms together in front of their chest. Help them find their balance by shifting their weight back and forth from foot to foot.

Invite the children to pretend they are frogs. Recite the frog rhyme a few times, and have children join in. They can hop around and croak. Encourage them to make a really big leap into the lake at the rhyme's end.

Frog rhyme

I am a happy frog

I live beside the bog

But when the sun begins to bake

I like to jump into the lake

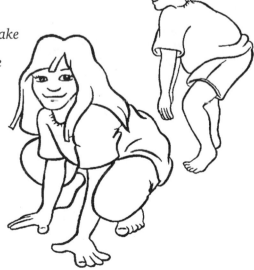

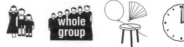

Lying Down, the Rest Position

Props: mats

♪ **Music:** background music (optional)

This simple pose is excellent for relaxation (see games 29–37 on pages 67–77).

Have the children lie on their backs. Ask them to bend their knees and wrap their arms around their legs, hugging the knees against the chest. If that is difficult, they can put their hands behind their knees, on the backs of their thighs. Invite children to rock forward and back, and side to side, in this position. This rocking motion massages the back and relaxes the muscles.

After a few minutes, have children release their knees and slide their legs out straight again. Tell them to keep the legs slightly apart.

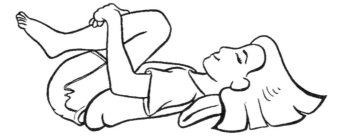

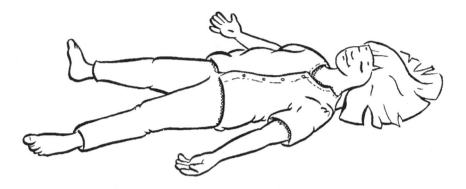

Then have children place their hands on their bellies or by their sides with hands open and palms upwards. Choose the hand position according to whether you want the children's attention directed inward or outward. When they lie down with their hands on their bellies, they can feel their breathing and stay in contact with themselves. With hands open at their sides, they are open to the world around them.

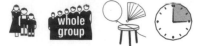

The Cat

Props: mats

♪ **Music:** background music (optional)

Crawling on hands and knees is very good for the back, making it supple and strong without putting any weight on it. And, of course, crawling around like an animal is loads of fun.

Invite the children to get down on their hands and knees and imagine they are cats. Ask if the children have ever seen Halloween decorations showing black cats arching their backs. Point out that cats often arch their backs to stretch and invite the children to stretch like cats. Encourage them to arch their backs, dropping their heads and stretching their backs up into a curve. Then ask children to curve their backs in the other direction, raising their heads and dropping their bellies so that their backs make a downward curve. Let children switch back and forth between the two positions a few times.

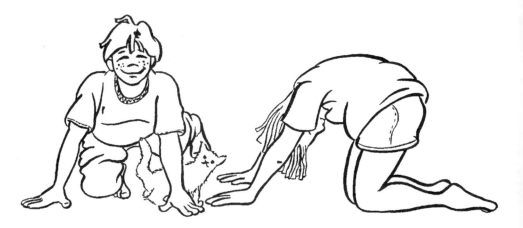

Next, invite them to stay on hands and knees and stretch one leg out straight behind them. Have them put that knee back down and stretch the other leg. After doing this a few times, ask children to stretch one arm out straight in front, then the other arm, and repeat a few times. Now challenge the children to stretch out one arm and the opposite leg at the same time (left hand and right leg or right hand and left leg). This might not be suitable for preschoolers. Tell them: "Think about your other hand and knee that are still on the ground. They are supporting you and need to be strong so you don't fall. Keep them firmly planted on the ground." Have them switch sides and stretch the other arm and the other leg. Then children can repeat the exercise a few times.

After the children have done their cat stretches, invite them to play for a while as cats. The children can crawl around the room, imitating cat noises and movements. They might meow, purr, hiss, growl, curl up for a nap, drink by lapping with their tongues, give themselves a bath, or chase a mouse. You could guide them in their play, or let them make up their own actions.

Variations:

- Encourage older children to coordinate the cat stretch with their breathing. The children can switch back and forth between the two positions as they breathe in and out. On the exhale, have them drop their heads and arch their backs. On the inhale, have them raise their heads and drop their bellies so that their backs make a downward curve.

- Before the children try stretching out opposite arms and legs, have them stretch out one side and then the other. First they might stretch out their right arm and their right leg, then their left arm and their left leg.

- Invite a volunteer to lead the others in imitating cats. The volunteer can call out suggestions about how to move—play with a ball of string, take a bath, and so on.

23

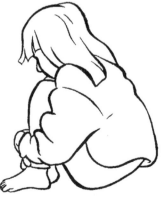

Back Roll, Rag Doll, and Plow

Props: mats

♪ **Music:** background music (optional)

Children love swings and rocking horses, with good reason: The rocking movement creates harmony and relaxation. In this game they can become their own swing. The exercise stretches the back and spine, keeping them flexible. Folding the abdomen inwards stimulates the circulation around the abdominal organs. The exercise also stretches the muscles at the back of the legs, muscles that tend to be short and tight, even in young children. Most important, the children really enjoy themselves.

Make groups of five to nine children. Have each group stand in a circle and hold hands. Ask them to keep holding hands as they sit, then lie down with their feet pointing toward the center. Invite each group to imagine that the circle is a wheel, with their bodies as the spokes and their arms as the tire. Have them close their eyes just for

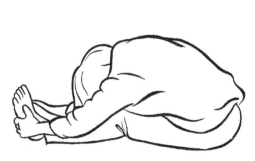

rag doll pose   **ball pose**

a minute and imagine that the wheel is turning, slowly at first, and then quickly.

Now ask the children to slowly raise and gently lower their legs, one after the other. Encourage them to synchronize the movement, watching their neighbors and trying to move at the same time. Have them repeat the movement five times. Next, have children raise both their legs together and gently bring them down again together, repeating five times. Now have them raise one leg until it is pointing straight up in the air and hold it there while they bring the other leg to meet it. Tell them that the ring of legs looks like the candles on a birthday cake. Ask them to dip their legs down a little and raise them back up again, repeating five times. Have them place their hands on their bellies as they do this, and point out how hard the belly muscles become. Now have them dip their legs to the left and back up, repeating three times. Do the same exercise dipping the legs to the right.

Invite children to bend their knees and roll up into a sitting position. Tell them not to force it: If rolling doesn't work, they should just sit up. Then ask children to sit with their legs together, stretched out straight in front. (See the staff pose on page 42.) Invite them to imagine they are all soft and floppy, like a rag doll. Tell them to flop forward over their legs. (See illustration of the rag doll pose on page 50.) If it feels comfortable, the children could rest their heads on their knees and hold their feet with their hands. Remind them not to push their bodies into positions that hurt. As children are flopped forward, encourage them to notice where their bodies move as they breathe. After a minute, have them sit up slowly. Seated again, have them lean to the left and to the right, repeating three times.

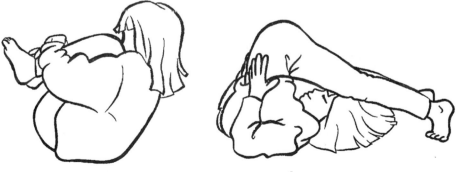

back roll   **plow pose**

Now have children bend their knees and curl up into a ball, putting their heads down and wrapping their arms around their knees. (See illustration of the ball pose on page 50.) Invite children to roll back in this position, and then rock forward again. (See illustration of the back roll on page 51.) Tell them to roll forward back at their own speed. If they need to rest, they can pause while sitting up or while rolled back.

Next, have them try rolling like this but with the legs straight. If they roll forward, they will be in the rag doll position again. If they roll all the way back, they will be in the plow position. (See illustration of the plow position on page 51.) Children may want to use their arms to support their backs while they pause in the plow position. They can hold this pose for a while, or go back to rolling forward and back. The rag doll posture and the plow can be seen as the two extreme points of the back roll and flow from the rocking movement. Children literally roll into the rag doll and the plow postures. Let children explore these movements for 3–6 minutes.

Finally, have children lie for 30 seconds with eyes closed and focus on how their bodies feel. Ask them to stand up slowly, hold hands, and hop towards the middle of the circle and back out again, then repeat. Then have them walk to the middle, raise their arms, and slowly walk backwards. Ask them to sit down and discuss what the exercise was like.

Variations:

- In all three exercises (back roll, rag doll, and plow) the children can keep their legs spread apart and hold their feet with their hands.

- In this description the series of exercises is done in a circle. This encourages cooperation. The children will see that when working together they create interesting shapes that they would not be able to do alone. Of course all the exercises can be done individually or spread around the room. The advantage in that case would be that the children can concentrate more on their individual work since they don't need to keep an eye on the others.

The **Cobra**

Props: mats

In this posture the front of the body is expanded and opened. This gives a feeling of power and it strengthens the back and the whole upper body. Make sure that the children do the posture correctly, and don't arch their backs too far. Since the back is very delicate, it is important for children to learn the correct way of moving at a young age.

Ask the children to lie down on their bellies. Invite them to feel the floor beneath them and the air around them. Before they begin the pose, remind them that it is very important to move gently, and not to force the body to stretch too far. You might instruct them as follows:

This pose is called the cobra, which is a kind of snake. Have you ever seen a snake raising its head up to strike? We are going to rise up like cobras. Put your hands palm-down on the floor, under your shoulders.

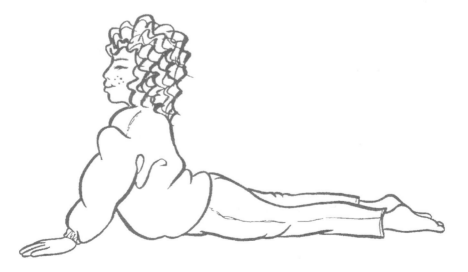

Slowly and gently raise your head and then pull your chest forward and up using your belly and back muscles. Your belly gets hard so your back is not curved too far. Push your feet and the area below your belly button into the floor. Use your hands to help keep your balance, not to push yourself up farther. Don't bend backwards. Stretch your head forward and up, away from your shoulders. Now slowly and gently lower yourself to the floor.

You should follow this pose with the child's pose (see game 27 on page 59), to rest the children's backs.

Variations:

- Invite children to curl their tongues up to the roof of their mouths as they hold the pose, imitating the body's lifted position.

- When the children are in the cobra posture, they can make a hissing sound like a snake.

The
Grasshopper

Props: mats

This posture stretches the front of the body and strengthens the back muscles. It also stimulates the organs and improves circulation. As children hold the pose, make sure they focus on using the abdominal muscles; this is necessary to support the back.

Have the children lie down on their bellies. Invite them to feel their breathing, the floor beneath them, and the air around them. Have them place their hands together in front of their head, with their elbows out to the side and their forehead resting on their hands. You might instruct them as follows:

Imagine you are a grasshopper, with very long, powerful legs. Tighten up your belly muscles so that your belly becomes hard. Now raise one leg a little bit off the floor, stretching it up and behind you. Breathe in and out gently and become aware of how that feels in your body. When you are finished, put that leg down and raise the other leg.

You should follow this pose with the child's pose (see game 27 on page 59), in order to rest the children's backs.

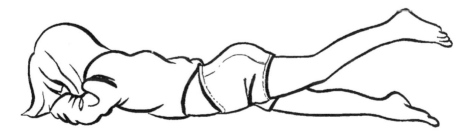

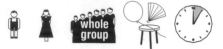

26

The Swan

Props: mats

The swan pose is a natural exercise for children. You can observe children as young as 2 grabbing one foot and pulling it up and backwards. This pose stretches the front of the body and gives a feeling of space. Children must open up the front of the body to hold the leg, rather than arching backward. The pose helps develop balance and self-confidence. The connection of hand and foot creates a circle and keeps the child in contact with herself.

Swans are beautiful birds. They radiate power as they swim silently or flap their enormous wings. Begin by telling the story of the ugly duckling, and then demonstrate the pose:

The cute yellow ducklings all tease the ugly gray duckling who looks so different. He leaves the farmyard and tries to make his way alone. Then one day, he sees swans flying overhead. He admires them so much he wants to be one of them. To his surprise, the swans accept him. When he sees his reflection in the water, he realizes that he has grown into a beautiful white swan.

Get down on your hands and knees. Imagine that you are a beautiful white swan, large, strong, and not afraid of anything. Make your belly hard—during this exercise it's important to keep your belly hard so that your back doesn't get too hollow. Lift your left leg off the ground and bend your knee so your left foot comes up. At the same time, reach your right

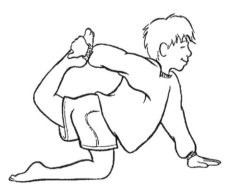

swan pose on hands and knees

hand behind you to grab your left foot. If you lose your balance, try it again more slowly. Your arm, leg, and body will form a big circle. Bend forward. Your head goes up as you move. Become aware of how your body feels. Be aware of the ground supporting you.

Have the children switch sides and try the pose again. You may want to follow this pose with the child's pose (see game 27 on page 59), to rest the children's backs.

Variations:

- While on hands and knees, have children grasp the foot on the same side instead of grasping the opposite foot. In other words, children will do the pose as described above, but grasp the left foot with the left hand and then the right foot with the right hand.

- Have the children stand. Remind them to keep their bellies hard, as described above. Invite them to lift their left leg behind them and at the same time reach their left hand back and grasp the left foot. Tell them to lean forward, stretching out the right hand for balance, and raise the left foot into the air. (See the illustration below.) Then have them repeat the pose on the right side.

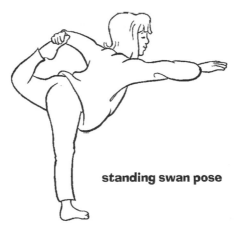

standing swan pose

- Invite the children to lie down on their right side, supporting their head with their right hand. Ask them to raise the left leg and bend the knee, and at the same time reach the left hand out until they can grab the left foot with the left hand. Have them raise the left foot up and back. (See the illustration below.) Repeat the stretch on the other side.

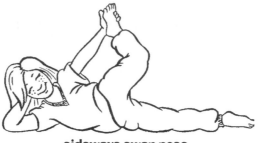

sideways swan pose

- Have the children lie on their bellies. Depending on their age and ability, have them do either a half bow or a full bow. For a half bow, the children bend one knee and reach behind them with the opposite hand to grasp the foot (i.e., right hand and left foot), then raise their chest and bent knee off the floor, forming a bow shape. For a full bow, the children bend both knees and reach behind them with both hands to grasp both feet. Challenge them to raise their knees and chest off the ground, arching to form a bow. (See the illustration below.)

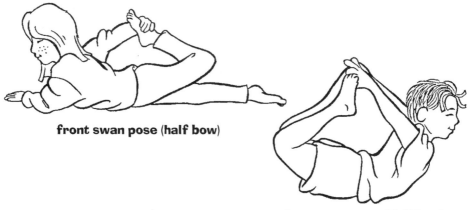

front swan pose (half bow)

front swan pose (full bow)

You should follow this pose with the child's pose (see game 27 on page 59), to rest the children's backs.

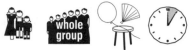

27

Child's Pose

Props: mats

This is a wonderful posture that gives a feeling of safety and privacy. It is a position in which a child can find peace. The child's pose is an excellent close to a yoga session. It should also be used after poses in which the back is arched backward, such as the cobra, the grasshopper, and the swan.

To begin, have children kneel with their big toes together, heels slightly apart. They should be sitting comfortably on their heels. Next, ask them to put their hands on the ground and roll forward until their foreheads come to rest between their hands. Remind them to keep their bottoms sitting on their heels. Tell them: "Your weight should be resting on your heels, not on your head. The head is a resting point, not a support."

Variations:

- Have children spread their knees slightly apart, giving the abdomen more space.

- Have children stretch their arms straight out in front.

- Have children lay their arms along their sides, pointing back toward the feet.

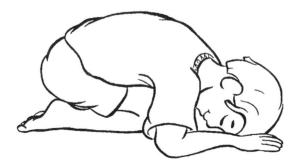

28

Sun Salutations
for Children

Props: mats

Most of us don't see the sunrise very often. There is something so magical about the moments when dawn begins to break, perhaps because without sunlight there would be no life on earth. We can recall that magical feeling through the sun salutation.

The salutation is a series of exercises linked together into a whole. It is a dance in which movement and rest alternate, a dance you can do quickly or slowly depending how you feel. The postures are not an end in themselves—the flow of movements, one into another, is the essence of the sun salutation.

The salutation gives the body more strength and suppleness. It is relaxing and at the same time enhances the flow of energy, improves the circulation, and invigorates the lymphatic system. The deep breathing cleanses the lungs. The breathing will come naturally with the movements: You don't need to draw children's attention to their breathing unless they are holding their breath.

This version of the salutation to the sun has been specially adapted for the delicate, young body. The children enjoy this exercise very much—they can really put their hearts into it. The entire body is exercised and any discomfort is quickly dissolved. After the salutation, they will be quiet and alert, nice and balanced.

In the process of teaching the children to do the salutation to the sun, use the following verse:

"Salutation to the Sun"

I make a circle nice and round
Now I stamp hard on the ground
I bend and walk my hands, then stop

Now I'm a triangle with my bottom on top
I'm a lion big and strong
Now I'm stretching lean and long
Other side
Now I hide
Here I am!
Now I stand
I spin willy-nilly
And try to look silly

While the children sit in a circle, tell them that they are going to learn a dance called a salutation to the sun. Explain that a salutation is a way of saying hello. Tell them a poem will help them remember the movements of the dance. Recite the poem a couple of times, then demonstrate the movements that go along with it. It is amazing how quickly children can learn something. After you demonstrate the salutation a few times, have the children spread out around the room.

Have them begin by standing with their hands in the prayer position (palms together at chest height). Lead the children in the sun salutation, pausing often the first time to explain each movement.

(Starting position)
Before they begin the movements, have the children take a second to imagine the sun. Tell them: "Close your eyes and in your mind see the sun shining brightly. It's just right: not too hot and not too cold."

I make a circle nice and round
Have the children trace the shape of a circle with their hands, sweeping their arms up above their heads and down to their thighs. This movement helps stretch the front of the body. The circle symbolizes the sun and the self as a complete being. Tell children: "Open your eyes and, with your arms, make big circles in the air. Look up towards the sun and feel the space around you."

Now I stamp hard on the ground
The children lift their feet one by one and stamp on the ground. This contact with the earth helps children feel balanced and self-assured. Ask them: "How does the ground feel? Is it hard? Is it soft?"

I bend and walk my hands, then stop
Now I'm a triangle with my bottom on top
The children should bend over at the waist with a straight back, touching their hands to the floor. Then they walk their hands forward while their feet stay in place. Encourage them to keep their backs straight. Their bodies will end up in a triangle shape, with their bottoms forming the top point. The two lower points of the triangle are the hands and feet on the ground. This position (known as "downward dog") stretches the back and the legs and strengthens the arms.

I'm a lion big and strong
Now the children bend their knees and go down on all fours. This line of the poem makes the children feel powerful.

Now I'm stretching lean and long
Still on all fours, have the children stretch their right arm out in front of them and their left leg straight behind them, as in game 22 on page 48 (The Cat). Encourage them to look upward.

Other side
Have the children switch sides and repeat the exercise above: They should stretch their left arm out in front of them and their right leg straight behind them, as in game 22 on page 48 (The Cat). Again, encourage them to look upward.

Now I hide
Ask the children to go into the child's pose (see game 27 on page 59), with their hands hiding their faces. Have them hold this pose for a moment. As children make themselves small, encourage them to feel the security and safety of this position; they should experience the feeling of being comfortable in their own skin and being supported by the earth.

Here I am!
Now the children come out of hiding. They should raise their heads and use their hands to push themselves up into a squatting position—see game 20 on page 45 (The Frog).

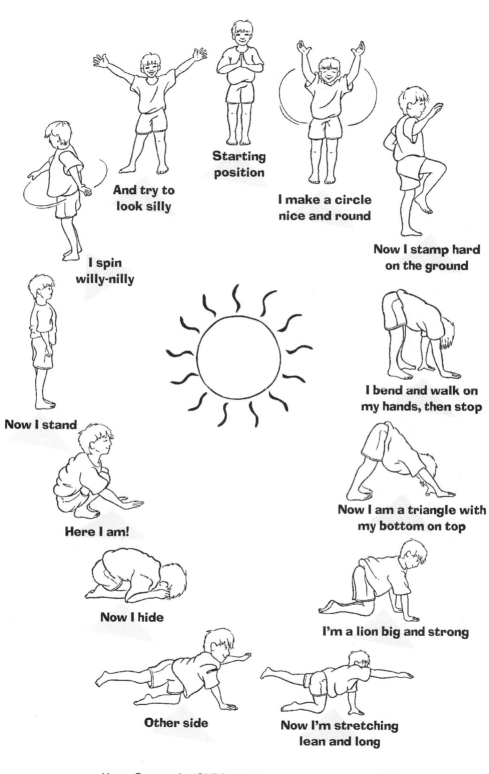

And try to
look silly

Starting
position

I make a circle
nice and round

Now I stamp hard
on the ground

I spin
willy-nilly

I bend and walk on
my hands, then stop

Now I stand

Now I am a triangle with
my bottom on top

Here I am!

Now I hide

I'm a lion big and strong

Other side

Now I'm stretching
lean and long

Now I stand
Ask the children to stand up tall, assuming the mountain pose (see game 17 on page 38). Alternating between big and small poses keeps the body supple.

I spin willy-nilly
Have the children stay on their spots, open their arms out wide, and turn in a clockwise circle. Spinning is energizing. Encourage the children to feel the space around them.

And try to look silly
When the children stop spinning, invite them to strike a silly pose of their own invention. Encourage them to make up any fun or strange position they like. Inventing a pose helps the children learn to value their own creative ideas. Being different is fine; acting silly can be great fun.

Now have children complete the cycle by bringing their hands together again in front of their chest. Repeat the salutation until the children have learned it and the movements begin to flow gracefully.

After about half an hour, gather the children into their circle again. Discuss the rhyme and the movements with them. Ask: "Which movements did you like best? Which did you not like? Can you tell us why?" Invite each child in turn to do his favorite movement, the one that felt best. Make a mental note of children's comments about the rhyme and consider making revisions next time based on these reactions. Finally, have the children lie down and play them some relaxing music.

Relaxation

This section is made up of short yoga exercises and guided fantasies to teach the children to relax and sit quietly.

In nature we see many phases and rhythms. With the change of seasons we see phases of growth and regeneration. We are also familiar with the rhythms of day and night that regulate our sleeping and waking cycles. Action and rest, tension and relaxation follow each other automatically. Both are needed for balance. In the West we divide the unity of ourselves into body and mind. In fact, they are irrevocably bound to each other. Both body and mind become relaxed in the relaxation exercises—busy thoughts float away and we let go of unnecessary movements.

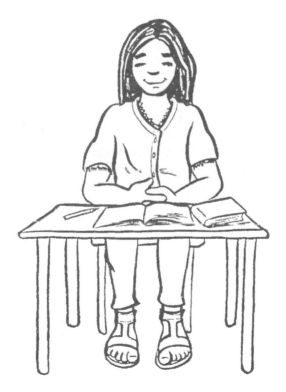

The breath is key to moving from tension to relaxation. To promote relaxation, we use slow belly breathing—the movement of the breath is low down in the abdomen, and controlled naturally by the diaphragm. For more information about breathing, see the section of breathing exercises and games on pages 14–36.

Make sure you establish the right atmosphere before starting a relaxation exercise. The room should be familiar, warm, not too bright, and quiet. When working with a brand-new group who don't know you or each other well, don't use relaxation exercises right away. The unknown creates tension. After a few classes, when the situation has become more familiar, relaxation exercises will become more suitable.

After relaxation exercises, it's important to ask each child about her experience and feelings. This teaches a child how to put her feelings into words so she becomes more conscious of these feelings. Even more important, each child should be listened to. Other children should not interrupt; they should hear each child out without making any comments. As leader, make the child feel as secure as possible and ask questions to help her gain more insight and understanding of the situation.

In the Classroom

Children today are under a good deal of stress. The school day is long and although there are pauses from physical effort, there is not enough real relaxation. Even elementary school children have a busy agenda with lots of appointments. When their day is done, children tend to lounge in front of the TV for distraction rather than finding a way to relax and unwind. These children tend to have more and more sleep problems.

The following exercises can be adapted for use in the classroom. Instead of sitting or lying on the floor, the children sit straight on their chairs with both feet planted firmly on the floor and hands on the belly or the knees, palms upward. The children enjoy this compulsory rest and it often changes their mood completely. When there is tension in the classroom, you can often diffuse it with one minute's silence instead of going into a lengthy discussion.

Shake It Loose

Props: mats

This game helps children learn to relax by giving them direct feed-back. One child lies on the floor and lets another child move his limbs around. The child who is lying relaxed on the floor can feel it if his limbs don't flop freely. The child who is moving the arm or leg can instantly feel any resistance. The children practice letting go of muscle tension and learn to trust each other.

Have the children work in couples. Marcus lies on his back on the mat with Shauna sitting next to him. Marcus tries to relax completely and Shauna puts both hands on his leg. First she lets the leg stay on the ground, but shakes it gently back and forth. If Marcus is really relaxed, then the leg and foot will roll freely. If this goes well, Shauna can lift the leg by grabbing the calf and shake it until the foot swings very loosely. She can then carefully move the leg around, making sure not to force anything. She must also be careful not to spoil the trust Marcus has in her—no sudden movements and don't drop that leg!

Partners can shake both legs and arms loose in this way. Take a few minutes for each limb, and then have partners switch roles.

Variation: Once the children have more experience they can also work in threes, fours, and fives. One child lies down and the other children take an arm or leg each.

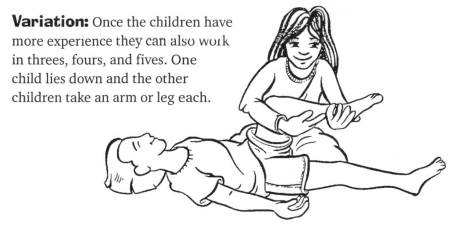

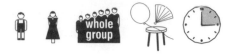

Being Heavy

Props: mats

When the body is relaxed it feels warm and heavy. By focusing on feelings of warmth and heaviness, we can help our bodies to relax. This relaxation exercise adapts for children the methods of Dr. Johannes Schulz's autogenic training. Once you have guided children through this simple exercise a few times, they will be able to do it by themselves. Encourage them to remember these techniques whenever they need to relax.

Have the children lie on their backs in the rest position (see game 21 on pages 46–47). Ask them to close their eyes and listen to your voice. Speak very quietly and slowly:

Let your thoughts go down to your feet. Feel how they are touching the floor. Where is the ground and where does the air begin? Can you feel it? Your feet are very warm and heavy. Feel how warm and heavy they are. Imagine that the sun is shining on your feet.

Moving from the feet up, go over every part of the body. Describe how warm and heavy each body part feels:

- calves/lower legs

- knees

- thighs/upper legs

- hips/bottom

- abdomen/belly

When you reach the abdomen, talk about the breath as well as about feelings of warmth and heaviness. Tell the children: "Feel how the breath makes your belly move up and down, like waves in the ocean. Feel your belly moving up and down, very gently and slowly."

Move up the body to:

- the back

- hands

- lower arms

- upper arms

- shoulders

- neck

Finally you reach the head. *Do not* tell the children that their heads feel warm: A warm head causes headaches and tension. Instead, tell them that the forehead is *nice and cool*. Tell them: "Imagine there is a soft, cool breeze blowing on your forehead. Your head feels heavy and your forehead is cool."

After you have talked about the head, let the children lie still for a few minutes. Then finish the exercise: "Very gently start to move your feet and hands. Breathe in more deeply and stretch out. Slowly sit up and tell us how it felt to relax your body this way."

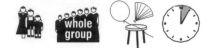

Sleep

Props: mats

♪ **Music:** relaxing music

This game gives children a chance to think about what sleep positions are most relaxing for them.

Have the children find a place to lie down on the floor. Tell them:

When you go to bed at night, do you like to lie on your side, your back, or your belly? Do you curl up or stretch out? Choose a comfortable position to go to sleep. Turn over if you need to so you can get really comfortable. Close your eyes and pretend you are going to sleep. Listen to the music and relax.

The first time younger children try this relaxation exercise, end it after a couple of minutes. With older children, you can extend it for as long as 10 minutes.

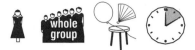

White Light

Props: mats

The whole body is addressed in this guided fantasy exercise. Positive thinking can create a positive feeling in the body.

Have the children sit or lie on the ground (see game 19 on pages 42–44 and game 21 on pages 46–47). Ask them to close their eyes, and instruct them as follows:

Feel your breathing becoming slow and regular. Put your attention on a spot above your head and imagine a white light shining there. The light can shine though the crown of your head and come inside you. The light flows into every part of your body. The light brings you energy and strength. It will make you feel stronger.

First you feel the white light in your head. Then it flows down into your throat, your chest, and your heart. You can feel the light in your shoulders. Now it flows down your arms to your fingers. If you feel tension in your body, let it flow away through your fingertips. Now you feel the white light flowing down your back and through your belly. Next it flows down your legs and right down to your feet. You can feel the white light flowing through your whole body. It makes you feel safe and warm. Your breathing is getting more and more relaxed.

The guided relaxation lasts about 5 to 10 minutes. After you finish talking, let the children lie there for a few more minutes. Then ask them to start moving gently and stretch out. Invite them to talk about their experiences of this relaxation exercise.

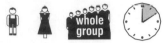

Energy in Your Hands

This game shows children how they can use concentration to bring energy to different parts of their bodies. Have the children sit in a circle on the floor (see game 19 on pages 42–44). Ask them to close their eyes and place their hands on their thighs with palms turned upwards. Then tell them:

Concentrate on your left hand and imagine that you are holding a small ball. That ball gives off warmth and energy. Feel the warmth going from your hand into your little finger, your ring finger, middle finger, index finger, and thumb. The warmth is going to flow from your hand into your wrist. Now you feel the warmth flowing from your wrist to your elbow, up your arm to your shoulder and your neck. Your left arm and your neck are now nice and warm. Keep the left hand warm.

You notice that the energy in your left hand has flowed all the way up your left side. Now concentrate on your right hand. There is a ball of energy in your right hand, too.

Again, name each finger in turn and go up the body as before. Then tell the children: "Your hands, arms, shoulders, and neck all feel lovely and warm. Now put your nice warm hands on whatever part of your body needs a little extra warmth." Through choosing where to place their hands, the children learn to give themselves what they need.

Pause for a few minutes while the children remain sitting or lying with eyes closed. Then ask them to open their eyes and discuss their experiences.

Variation: The same exercise can also be done with feet and legs. Ask the children to imagine that their legs are touching a warm blanket. Then name the toes and parts of the legs.

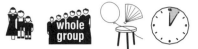

Rag Doll

Props: mats

Lying folded over their own laps gives the children a sense of security. This position helps them relax.

Have the children sit with their legs out in front of them (see game 19 on pages 42–44). Tell them:

Imagine that you are soft and floppy like a rag doll. First stretch your arms out and make yourself as tall as you can. Now bend forward as far as you can and let your upper body rest on your legs. Make your upper body as floppy as it can be. Your arms are also completely floppy. I'm going to come around and see if your arms are really floppy like a rag doll.

Go around the room and move one or both arms of each child. Then ask them to sit up again slowly. This takes several minutes.

Note: If the muscles at the back of the thighs are short, this pose can be painful for a moment. Any pain should go away immediately afterward. To prevent injury or discomfort, remind the children not to force their bodies into the pose.

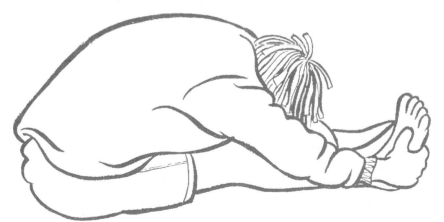

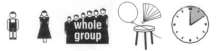

Tensing and Relaxing

Props: mats

If you ask people to relax a particular part of their bodies, their first reaction is often to tense that body part. It sounds ironic, but this initial tensing can aid in the relaxation. Tensing the part of the body they are trying to relax helps people to feel that part better. Then they can truly relax it. That is the principle on which this exercise is based.

Tell the children they can choose whether to lie down or sit for this relaxation exercise. Instruct them as follows:

Close your eyes and feel the movement of your breathing. Make a fist with your hand. Feel how strong and firm your fist can get. Feel the muscles of your upper arm tightening up. Hold that tension for a moment—and then let go. Relax all your fingers and let your arm hang loosely. Relax completely. We'll do that again. First make a firm fist, tighten up your arm, and then let go.

Now we will do the same thing with the other hand. Make a fist, feel how your arm tenses up as well, and then relax. Make a fist again, and relax your hand again. Now stretch your hands out, spreading the fingers, and be aware of how good this feels. Let your hands hang loose again. Notice how your hands and arms feel now.

Move on to the feet and legs, alternately tensing and relaxing them. When you are finished, tell the children: "Now that everything is so completely relaxed, become aware of how good that feels." Let the children remain in this relaxed position for a few minutes. Then ask them to stretch and sit up again and discuss how the exercise felt.

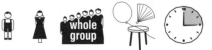

What Does Tension Feel Like?

Props: mats

One of the keys to relaxation is learning to recognize tension in the body. In this exercise, children tense parts of their bodies while other parts are relaxed. This gives them the chance to compare the feeling of tension and the feeling of relaxation. Once they can feel the difference between tension and relaxation, it becomes easier to relax.

Have children lie on their backs in the resting pose (see game 21 on pages 46–47). Lead them through a shortened version of game 30 on pages 68–69 (Being Heavy). Next, ask them to tense up one leg and slowly lift it a couple of inches off the ground, then slowly let it down again and rest for a moment. Have the children keep lifting and lowering the leg for a few minutes. Encourage them to notice what happens to their muscles and their breathing as they lift the leg up and down. Remind them to keep the other leg relaxed. Then tell them:

Be aware of how each leg feels. Can you feel a difference? Is one leg heavier, lighter, warmer, or colder than the other? Is one leg tingling? Does one leg feel longer than the other? Fatter or thinner? Maybe you don't feel any difference, or perhaps you feel something else. Think about how each leg feels.

Invite the children to sit in a circle and discuss how the exercise felt. Then switch legs and repeat the exercise.

Variation: The same exercise can be done with the arms.

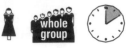

A Space of Your Own

The space surrounding our bodies belongs to us. If someone stands too close to us, we feel uncomfortable. Another person doesn't need to touch us for us to feel they have crossed our border. This exercise helps children claim their personal space and feel more self-assured.

Have the children spread out and find a place to sit or stand. Then ask them to close their eyes and tell them:

Feel where you are resting on the ground and where the ground is supporting you. If you are standing, plant your feet firmly on the ground. If you are sitting, feel how securely your body has come to rest. Today we are going to create a space of our own. Imagine that you are able to breathe in through every part of your body. You can't really do that, but we are going to pretend. While you're there with your eyes closed, nice and still, let your thoughts go to your head and breathe into the space above it. Create space for yourself, using your own energy. The space above you is yours; it belongs to you.

Now we do the same thing with the space in front of you. There is air in front of you, space that belongs to you. Breathe outward and feel how large you want that space in front of you to be. It can be as big as you like, but perhaps you'd like to keep it quite small.

Now we do the same behind us. Behind there is also space that belongs to you. Breathe into that space and make it your own. This makes you a bit bigger. We have space above us, in front of us, and behind us; now we have to make space at the sides. First on one side— there is space that belongs to you. Breath into that space. Now on the other side.

Feel the ground underneath you. That is also part of your space. Now you are in a bubble of space and you can feel the ground. This is your place on the earth, where you are safe. Make your bubble of space as large as you want it.

If you like, you can invite other people into your space in your mind. They come into your space, your place. Friends, brothers, sisters, your father, your mother... or maybe you don't want anyone in your space. It is your own space, so do what you like with it.

Let the children stay like this for several minutes. Then tell them: "You can keep that feeling of space around you. Breathe in deeply a couple of times. Now open your eyes and stretch your body."

Invite the children to discuss how the exercise felt, how big they made their space, and whether they invited anyone into their space. You might take this opportunity to discuss different ideas about personal space. Some people like a great deal of personal space, and want others to keep their distance. Other people are happy to sit close and like to touch when greeting. Help the children to understand that different people have different needs when it comes to space.

Sitting Still:
A Meditative Exercise

Meditation involves the letting go of conscious thought. When mind and body are relaxed, there are no active thoughts any more. Your mind stays on what is happening and how you feel. Children often find meditation exercises more natural than adults do. Children have fewer preoccupations and trains of thought to deal with. They are less apt to judge themselves and their inner feelings. This lack of preconception is essential for sitting still. Children are still able to be surprised and delighted to discover themselves, just as they are.

Always invite the children to talk about their experiences after a meditation exercise. It is important to know what is going on with the children. You can respond directly to children's thoughts, or make a note to address those issues in a future lesson.

If the children have practiced sitting still regularly over a longer period (perhaps twice a month for a year or so), you can gradually introduce themes for meditation. Games 39–43 on pages 81–85 cover themes that children come across in their daily lives, such as friendship, bullying, and anger. You could easily develop meditation exercises on other themes, such as families or fears.

When working with themes, your guidance is especially impor-tant. You need to be able to assess whether or not the children have been able to let go of judgement. Even more important: As leader, you yourself must not be judgmental about the children's feelings. It is not always easy to give a child this space if he has done things that you feel are wrong. Bullying is a good example. If, after going through the meditation exercise in game 40 on page 82 (Sitting Still and Bullying), a child admits to having bullied another child, you must listen without scolding or lecturing. You might say something like: "It's good that you've told us this. It probably wasn't easy. How does it feel now that you've told us? How do you feel about the child you bullied (hit, teased)? What would you like to do?"

Create an atmosphere in which all the children are welcome, even the children who behave or have behaved badly. The children need to know that they are accepted unconditionally. You do not need to approve of their behavior, but the children will never express their feelings if they have the feeling they are being judged. Be kind to the children and give them space so that they will be able to change their behavior. In this context, the children should not be forced to defend their behavior, should not be afraid of punishment, and should not be made to feel inferior or guilty. Guilt feelings do not necessarily lead to a change in behavior. The children can make mistakes in order to learn from them.

In the Classroom

All of these exercises can be used in an ordinary classroom with virtually no adaptation necessary. The themed meditations are especially useful for dealing with interpersonal issues in the classroom.

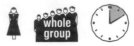

Sitting Still

Have the children sit comfortably with their backs straight and eyes closed. They could sit in a lotus or half-lotus position, or simply with their legs crossed (see game 19 on pages 42–44). Ask them to place their hands on their thighs or knees with palms facing upward, thumb and forefinger forming a circle. Touching thumb and fore-finger symbolizes being in touch with yourself. The other three fingers are stretched open, representing being open to anything the future brings. The children can also put their hands on their abdomens to stay closer to themselves. Tell them:

Feel the ground (or chair) you are sitting on. Feel how strong it is and how it supports you. Breathe normally and observe the breath and the movements it makes in your body. Let your thoughts come and go like the clouds across a blue sky. They come and float away again by themselves. Try not to judge anything as good or bad, right or wrong. Maybe lots of thoughts will come to you and maybe none at all.

Let children sit for 5 to 10 minutes. Then invite them to talk about what it was like to sit still, and what went through their minds.

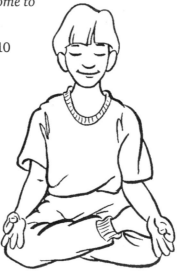

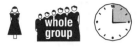

Sitting Still and Friendship

Children can form friendships at a very young age. A childhood friendship could last for an afternoon at the playground, or it could last a lifetime. Children can learn the value of friendship through play.

Have children sit with eyes closed as described in game 38 on page 80 (Sitting Still). Instruct them as follows:

While you are sitting, try not to think, but observe whatever thoughts come. You probably have a friend, or maybe there's someone you want to be friends with. Look at that friendship from a distance. What are the good things about friends? What are the things about friends that are not so good?

Let children sit for several minutes. Then ask them to open their eyes and invite them to share their thoughts about friendship. You might tell them:

You can get a lot out of friendship. You can laugh, play, and talk with your friends. You can help each other, and cheer each other up if you feel sad. Sometimes there can be problems in a friendship, too. You and a friend may not want to play the same games. You might hurt each other's feelings with things you say or do. When you have problems with friends, talk with them. Try to be honest and always say what you feel. Maybe you can work out a solution that would make you both happy. If you can't solve a problem, tell someone you trust—one of your parents or an older brother or sister or someone else.

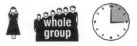

Sitting Still and **Bullying**

From a very young age children may take out their frustrations on other children. Bullying takes so many different forms—not only physical violence, but also malicious teasing, name-calling, and deliberate exclusion. It is so common, and in many cases the children are not aware of how hurtful it can be.

Bullying can be a big problem at school, but fortunately many schools have programs to prevent and alleviate bullying. When dealing with groups of children, it is important to draw attention to this issue now and then.

Have children sit with eyes closed as described in game 38 on page 80 (Sitting Still). Tell them:

Try not to think but just observe what comes into your head. Bullying means trying to hurt someone. Sometimes people bully by hitting, pushing, or kicking. Other people bully by teasing someone in a mean way to try to hurt their feelings. At some time in your life someone has probably tried to bully you. How did that feel? Have you ever bullied someone else? How did that feel?

Let the children sit for a few minutes. Then ask them to open their eyes and discuss their thoughts. The important thing is to remain as neutral as possible so that the children have the courage to speak openly about their feelings. You might tell the children:

Did you ever tell someone who was teasing you how bad it felt? Try to do that if it happens again. Also, watch what you do yourself. Maybe at some time you bullied someone and you feel a bit sorry about it now. Maybe you would like to tell that person that you will try not to do it again. If you are embarrassed to say it to the person's face, say it inside yourself now.

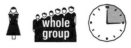

Sitting Still
and Beauty

"Who do you think is the prettiest?" a 4-year-old girl once asked me. Children learn very early to compare who they are and what they have with those around them: big, bigger, biggest; good, better, best. "I'm the oldest; I want to be first. Mine is the best; yours is ugly," they say to each other.

Self assurance comes from within, and so does beauty. This exercise helps children understand that it isn't necessary to compare themselves with other people. They all have their own beauty.

Have children sit with eyes closed as described in game 38 on page 80 (Sitting Still). Tell them:

Sit quietly and try not to think. Just watch what comes into your head. You are beautiful. It's not clothes that make you beautiful or ugly. You are always beautiful even if you think you look ugly. You are not more beautiful than anyone else. You may be beautiful in a different way, but that is not important. What is important is that you know you are beautiful on the inside and on the outside.

Let the children sit for a few minutes. Then ask them to open their eyes and share their ideas.

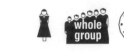

Sitting Still
and Anger

Anger creates tension in the body. If someone is angry and doesn't find an outlet for those feelings, the constant muscle tension can cause physical problems, usually pain. Letting go of anger can be a huge relief. In order to make this possible we first teach the children to be aware of their feelings.

Have children sit with eyes closed as described in game 38 on page 80 (Sitting Still). Tell them:

Sit quietly and try not to think. Just observe what comes into your mind. Do you sometimes feel angry? Where in your body do you feel that?

This part of the exercise should be very short: The object of this exercise is not to create or imagine anger. The children need only a few moments to feel any anger that is inside them. Then ask them to open their eyes and tell about their experiences.

Ask each child, "When you are angry, where do you feel it in your body? What could you do to let the anger out safely?" If a child says, "I feel it in my legs, but I don't know what I want to do," you might suggest that the child stamp on the floor. There are a number of activities you can use as an outlet for the anger—yelling, running, jumping, punching the air, and so on.

Once the children recognize their feelings, they can give feelings of anger a place. If they want to, they can express the anger in order to relax and be happy. The important thing is to make it clear that anger is not wrong. If children want to hang on to their anger, that's okay.

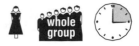

Sitting Still
and Happiness

Being happy with yourself and being happy with your situation is something children can learn. Happiness is connected with self-confidence and daring to express your happiness. Just like anger, happiness is an emotion that is reflected in the body. Being conscious of feelings can help children to choose or avoid these emotions.

Have children sit with cyes closed as described in game 38 on page 80 (Sitting Still). Tell them:

As you sit still, try not to think, but simply to observe whatever comes into your mind. Imagine that you are very happy. How do you feel in your body when you are happy? What makes you happy? Are you happy with yourself?

Let the children sit for a few minutes. Then ask them to open their eyes and discuss their experiences.

Cooperation and Trust Games

This section contains games that teach children to work together and trust each other through play. If people trust you and dare to show their vulnerability, it gives a wonderful feeling and makes you feel responsible for them. If you have trust in others, you can dare to show your feelings and weaknesses. You no longer need to keep defending yourself because you are more likely to be protected by the others than hurt by them. *You can be yourself!* This means that you aren't afraid to say no if you don't yet feel comfortable with a particular exercise. Knowing your own limitations and respecting others' boundaries is part of the learning process in the games that follow.

Without an atmosphere of trust it is best not to do trust games. This sounds paradoxical, since trust exercises might seem to be exactly what is needed in that situation. When children are afraid, you need to be very careful and sensitive towards which trust games you can safely do and which not. It is essential to build up trust step-by-step. In choosing trust games, the ages of the children are not terribly important, but the feelings of responsibility on one side and trust on the other are vital. The trust children put in each other must not be betrayed.

It is always important to discuss yoga games with the children afterward, but this is especially true with trust games. Use the children's feedback to adjust the games to the correct maturity level for the children in the group.

In the Classroom

These days children engage in a huge variety of activities on an individual basis. They sit by themselves behind a computer. They watch TV—perhaps together with other people, but each in a private world. Schools emphasize grades and performance; the children learn to compare themselves with others and to be competitive. Some even try to look better by belittling others. Children can be quite vicious towards each other without even realizing it. Unfortunately, bullying is a common problem.

The classroom is a perfect place for children to develop trust in each other. The trust games that follow are equally suitable for the classroom, playground, gym, or yoga room.

Seeing-Eye Guide

Props: blindfolds for half the children (optional)

In this game, one partner is blindfolded, and the other acts as a guide. The different roles in this trust game are very easy to see: One partner must trust, and the other must take responsibility. The blindfolded partner is vulnerable and learns to trust the other. The guide has a protective role and is responsible for ensuring that the blindfolded partner doesn't bump into anything.

Divide the group into pairs. One partner should put on a blindfold or close his eyes. The other partner is the guide and walks carefully around the room. The blindfolded partner holds the guide by the elbow or lower arm. Holding an elbow or arm rather than being led around by the hand gives the blindfolded partner more confidence. He is following the guide rather than being steered by the guide. This lets the blindfolded partner retain a certain amount of independence and decreases the feeling of powerlessness.

The guide can say in advance what she plans to do—for example: "I'm moving a little to the right because there's a table and chair in the way. Now we're coming to the blackboard and we're going to walk along the wall."

Have partners switch roles. Changing roles between the blindfolded partner and the guide allows both children to experience being vulnerable and protective. This gives a feeling of equality.

Afterward discuss how the game went.

Variations:

- The guide doesn't speak and uses only body movements to lead the other.

- The guide takes the blindfolded partner by the hand and leads her around. Talk about the difference between this and guiding by the elbow.

45

Two Guides

Props: blindfolds for one-third of the children (optional)

In this game, two guides lead a blindfolded player. Cooperation and shared responsibility are important themes in this game. This game is easier for the blindfolded player than game 44 on page 88 (Seeing-Eye Guide), since she is less reliant on one person.

Divide the group into teams of three: one blindfolded player and two guides. (If blindfolds are not available, those players can close their eyes instead.) The blindfolded player takes the two guides by the elbow or lower arm (see game 44). The guides learn to guide the blindfolded player sensitively and also learn to work together. Have team members switch roles twice, so everyone has a turn in the middle.

Variation: Put some obstacles in the way so that the blindfolded player has to be guided over, around, or under them.

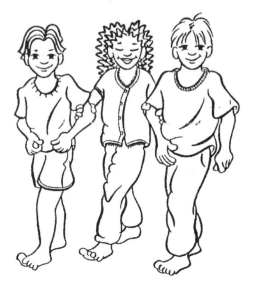

Dancing Together

Props: blindfolds for half the children (optional)

♪ **Music:** relaxing music

This game could be played as a sequel to game 44 on page 88 (Seeing-Eye Guide). Have the children form pairs and hold hands. One partner should wear a blindfold or close his eyes. The other partner moves to the music and leads the dance, without speaking. The blindfolded partner tries to be sensitive to the other's movements and join in the dance. Keep the music gentle.

The music provides a rhythm and makes the children want to move. This makes the movements more graceful. The blindfolded partner will learn to listen more closely to the music and to adapt to the partner's movements. The dancing partner should try to indicate with gestures and movements how she wants to dance: go forward, backward, slower, quicker, and so on.

Have partners change roles and dance again.

Variations:

- The dancing partner can use words to explain to the blind-folded partner what she wants to do.

- When the children have become comfortable with this style of dancing, put on faster music.

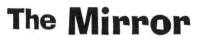

The **Mirror**

In this game, partners touch hands and mirror each other. The physical contact intensifies the element of cooperation in this mirror game. Partners need to concentrate and be careful about their movements.

Have pairs of children stand face-to-face and put their palms against the palms of their partner. One child is standing in front of the mirror and the other is the reflection. One child makes movements with her hands and the reflection follows. The hands must remain in contact.

Variations:

- The reflection closes his eyes.

- Both partners close their eyes.

- The children sit on the floor and touch feet.

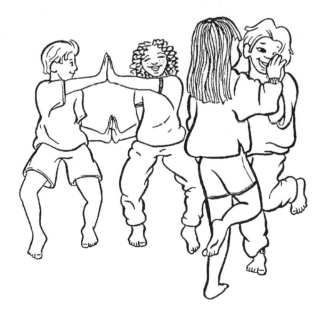

Walking Backward

In this game, one partner walks backwards while the other coaches him. We don't have eyes in the back of our heads, so some children find walking backwards quite difficult and even a bit scary. Children must rely on their partners to keep them safe. In addition to trust, this game develops coordination and awareness of space.

Divide the group into pairs. One child stands against a wall but faces the interior of the room while the other child faces the opposite wall and has her back to her partner. The walking partner must cross the room walking backward, without looking where she is going. The other partner watches the walker and guides her verbally: "I'm watching you, Annie; you're doing fine. Now move a little to your left; otherwise you'll bump into Tyrone."

Then have partners switch roles and play the game again.

Variations:

- The backwards walker keeps his eyes closed as he walks.

- Both the guide and the walker walk backwards across the room. The guide goes in front and is allowed to look over her shoulder periodically to see how far they still have to go.

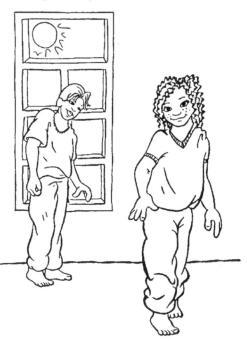

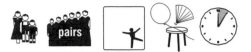

Jumping Together

Props: a long rope

Stretch the rope across the floor. Divide the group into pairs and have them hold hands. Pairs should line up and jump over the rope two by two.

    Because the children are holding hands, they have to cooperate to jump over the rope. They have to be aware of each other so they don't pull each other over. Partners must coordinate their efforts and jump at the same time. A child who is somewhat afraid can be positively encouraged by the energy and strength of his partner.

Variations:

- With older players, tie the rope to two objects or have volunteers help you hold it up to ankle or knee level. It will be more of a challenge to jump.

- Place two ropes on the ground a short distance apart. The pairs must jump over both ropes.

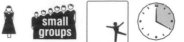

Circle of Friends

Divide the group into teams of six to ten children. Each team should stand close together in a circle with hands at chest height, palms towards the center of the circle. The circle should be about five feet in diameter. One child, Marisa, stands in the center. Tell the others to be ready to catch Marisa if she falls in their direction. They should not grab at her, but gently push her back toward the center with open hands. Ask Marisa to plant her feet firmly on the ground, stiffen her body, and let herself fall in whatever direction she chooses. The hands catch her and gently push her in the other direction. Marisa remains completely stiff, letting herself be pushed back and forth and supported by the hands of the other children. Make sure that the other children are always ready to catch her. After a few minutes, give another player a chance to take her place. Keep playing until everyone has a turn in the center.

This exercise requires close cooperation by all the children in the circle. They have to watch attentively because they have to work together to catch Marisa and move her to the center again. Marisa has to trust the others completely—she must trust their ability to catch her, their attention to her movements, and their care— otherwise she is not going to let herself fall freely.

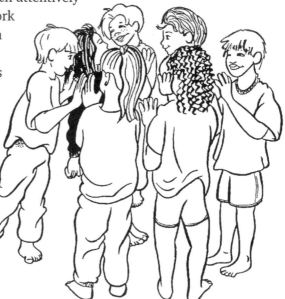

Lean
on Me

Divide the group into pairs with similar heights. Have partners sit on the floor back-to-back. Tell them that they will work together to stand up with their backs still touching. They must not come apart, and their hands cannot touch the ground. Point out that partners will have to use each other's backs as support. Now tell them to give it a try.

Partners can't see each other and must rely on feeling the other person's movement to know what to do themselves. This game requires true cooperation.

Variations:

- As they sit back-to-back, players put their arms and palms at their sides so that they are touching their partner's arms and palms. Pairs must keep their arms and palms touching (as well as their backs) while they stand up.

- Once pairs are standing upright, they can begin to walk sideways. Their backs (and arms if using that variation) should remain in contact.

^A Massage

Props: mats or towels

Massage relaxes both the giver and the receiver of the massage. The massage technique known as "hand over hand" is a simple, soft, stroking massage that is very simple to do. You place the first hand on the body and stoke downwards. You place the second hand more or less on the same point and follow the same stroking movement. Then you lift the first hand over the second hand and put it down in the original place again or slightly lower. This way you can massage down the body using both hands in turn in circular movements.

First demonstrate the massage on a volunteer. The volunteer lies on his belly on a mat or towel. Before you begin, rub your hands together to warm them up.

Kneel down close to the volunteer and place your hands low down on his back. Point out to the other children that you can feel his breathing through his back. Then put one hand between the shoulder blades and the other on the sacrum (in the center of the lower back, just above the buttocks) for about one minute. The volunteer will feel your hands high on the spine and low down, so he becomes more aware of his whole spine. This is very relaxing.

Bring both hands low down on the back and work your way up the spine and down the sides again using stroking movements. Then go hand over hand along the whole body—the back, top of the shoulders, upper arms, lower arms, and hands, and then down the back to the thighs, calves, and feet. Show the other children how the hand over hand technique works.

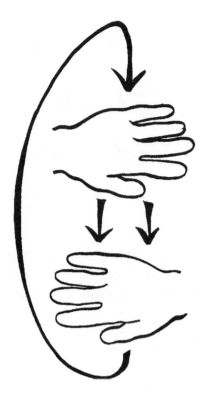

Now divide the group into pairs and have partners take turns massaging each other.

Note: Be sure to check on and follow your school or organization's policies on touching before introducing this exercise.

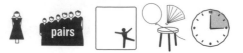

Stick Together

Props: a small stick or new, unsharpened pencil for each pair of children

Have pairs of children stand facing each other. Partners should hold out one hand to each other, palm facing forward. Place a stick between the hands of each pair. Partners must work to hold the stick together between their open palms, without grasping it.

When the sticks are steady, invite pairs to move around the room. One partner leads the movements and the other follows. Then leader and follower can switch roles.

This game requires patience and alertness from both children. They also need good coordination to hold the stick between them. It is great fun trying to keep the stick from falling.

Variations:

- Have the players close their eyes.

- Place the stick between the players' bellies instead of their hands (see illustration).

- Give each pair two sticks to balance, one for each hand.

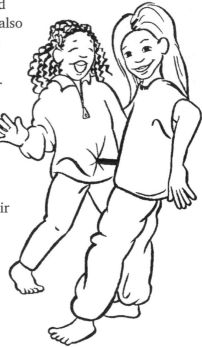

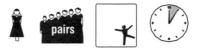

Lost
and Found

Have pairs of children stand face-to-face with eyes closed. Ask them to bring their hands up to chest height, slowly and carefully, so that they don't accidentally hit their partners. Encourage the children to concentrate on their hands: Do they feel warm or cold?

Now ask players to stretch their hands forward a little. Ask: "Can you feel the warmth of your partner's hands?" Have them move their hands forward until they bump into their partner's hands. Ask partners to put their palms together and hold them there. Then have pairs slowly bend their knees a little and come back up together.

Keeping their eyes closed, players should pull their hands back and turn around three times on the spot, coming back to face their partner. Challenge them to stretch out their hands again and find their partner's hands. Encourage players to do this without talking or opening their eyes. They will have to feel and listen carefully.

The children need cooperation and trust for this exercise to work. They learn to feel a person's presence and energy. Don't let players flail about carelessly. Players must reach for each other slowly and cautiously—otherwise one of them could get hurt.

Variations:

- Vary the level of difficulty by having the players make more or fewer turns before reaching out to find their partner.

- Have pairs make other movements together. They might do more knee bends, or raise their arms together.

Lessons with a Theme

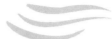

The games that follow are designed as complete yoga lessons, lasting about one hour each. Each one offers a range of activities: awareness, breathing, poses, movement, and relaxation. In these lessons, play and exercise blend into each other—pleasure is always an important component. They can be used just as described, or you can adapt them to your own purposes by using parts of them, adding your own variations, and combining lessons. Some of the lessons incorporate games from the earlier sections of the book. The themed lessons should serve as examples of how to construct unified lessons from these shorter games.

The four seasons—spring, summer, autumn and winter—are favorite themes. The children find it easy to relate to the seasons and will be able to contribute plenty of imagination to the class. As the seasons progress, the world is transformed again and again, offering an ever-changing feast for the senses. The seasons are children's first introduction to the cyclic nature of life.

Other subjects and special occasions can also be used as themes. Celebrations, and even sad subjects, allow children to give their emotions a place in their lives.

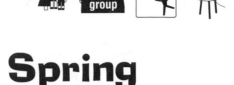

Spring

Props: mats, red and blue ribbons, flowers

In springtime, nature awakens: Seeds burst into life, buds become flowers. The birds return from their winter homes and our winter clothes go back into the closet. The world and all its inhabitants are full of energy and new life.

This yoga lesson takes these aspects of spring as inspiration for different kinds of movements, sounds, and cooperation exercises. The point of cooperation exercises is to show that the whole is greater than the sum of its parts: The children discover that they can sometimes do more together than they can independently.

Have the children form a circle and lie down on the floor. While they relax, sing (or recite) them this song about a seed:

Seed

Music: D. Bersma

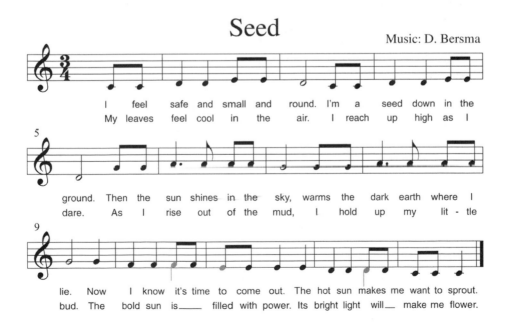

I feel safe and small and round. I'm a seed down in the
My leaves feel cool in the air. I reach up high as I

ground. Then the sun shines in the sky, warms the dark earth where I
dare. As I rise out of the mud, I hold up my lit - tle

lie. Now I know it's time to come out. The hot sun makes me want to sprout.
bud. The bold sun is____ filled with power. Its bright light will__ make me flower.

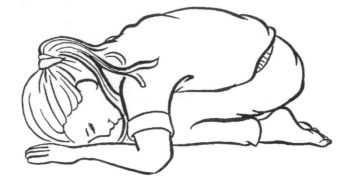

Ask the children to sit up, still in a circle. Show them how to go into the child's pose (see game 27 on page 59), kneeling with the forehead on the ground. Now invite them to act out the song:

Imagine that you are a seed. This is a good and safe feeling, nicely tucked inside yourself. While you are curled up like a seed, you will notice your head becoming warm. The sun warms your head and you lift it a little, but soon you relax it again because it's not warm enough yet. The sun shines down some more and you lift your head again a little higher. You look to left and right, feeling the sun's warmth.

Sit up now, but remain sitting on your heels. Bring your hands together in front of your chest. Open them slowly, like a flower opening. For a moment your wrists touch. Then open your arms wide like a big flower. Raise your arms and reach up toward the sun. Stretch for a moment. Now bring your arms down again.

Have the children act out the song again while you sing it (or recite it). Afterward, the children should still be kneeling in a circle, sitting on their heels. Tell them:

Now greet the sun together. Hold hands with the children on either side of you and as you breathe in, raise your arms towards the sun. Lower them again as you breathe out. (Repeat a few times.) Stand up so you are closer to the sun. Now do the greeting again. Hold hands; breathe in and raise your arms, then breathe out and lower them.

Repeat a few times and then invite the children to drop their hands and spread out around the room. Tell them:

Everyone has become a beautiful flower. Show us what kind of flower you are. You can do this standing still, but perhaps you can also walk like a flower. Now stand and look at all the other flowers.

This first part of the lesson lasts about 15 minutes. Next the children sit with their eyes closed and with hands on their bellies. This is a meditation exercise on flowers. You can ask the children to bring flowers to class with them, or you can bring flowers yourself and have each child choose one. Alternatively, you can simply have children picture flowers in their minds. Encourage them to experience the flowers (real or imagined) with all their senses:

Close your eyes and think about the flower in front of you (or picture a flower in your head). Can you see the flower in your mind? What color is it? What does it smell like? What is its shape? What are its petals like?

Invite the children to describe their flowers. Then continue with movement and sound exercises. Tell them:

Gently stand up and walk around the room. You are in a beautiful garden filled with flowers. When I clap, stand still and bend your knees so you can look at the flowers close up. There is a bee on the flower. Make the same sound as the bee: bzzzzz. (Repeat about six times.) If you put your hands over your ears and make the bzzzz sound again, you will hear it vibrating in your head.

Next, bring the children back into their circle for the cooperation exercise. Tell them:

Sit down with your legs pointing toward the center of the circle. Now lie on the ground with your legs apart. Put your feet against the feet of the children on either side of you, one against the foot of the person on your right and one against the foot of the person on your left. This way you form one big flower.

Tie each pair of feet together with ribbon, alternating red and blue (see illustration on page 103). Guide the children to raise and lower their legs as follows. Make sure they exhale as they lower the legs—this will help them use their abdominal muscles better. Tell them:

Breathe in, and as you breathe out, raise the foot that has the blue ribbon tied to it. Breathe in again and lower the foot gently when you breathe out.

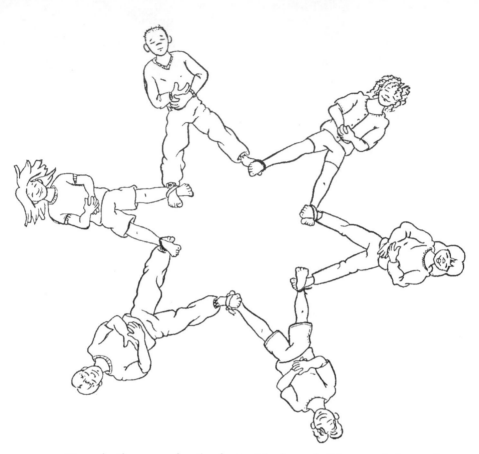

Now do the same for the foot with the red ribbon and then raise both legs at the same time. Afterward, invite the children to relax in their places, lying on their backs. End the lesson with the following story about flowers:

The weather is warm and sunny. Imagine you are in a field with colorful flowers all around you. They have a wonderful smell. You feel very happy here in this field. You decide to pick a big bunch of flowers. In your mind, pick the flowers. You want to give the flowers to someone special. Think about who you would like to have your flowers. (Pause for a minute so they can think of someone.) *Give the flowers to the person you chose.*

After they have lain still for a few minutes, untie the ribbons and invite the children to stretch out and yawn. Ask them what kind of flowers they picked, who they gave them to, and what the person said to them in response.

Summer

Props: rope

In the summer we love to go to the beach and enjoy the sun, the sand, and the sea. Most children enjoy water; they feel free and can move very easily in the water. Nonetheless, there are some children who are afraid of water and of the big, cold, deep ocean in particular. This lesson helps children learn to overcome their fears through discussion and pretend play.

Ask the children to lie on their backs, close their eyes, and picture a beach: warm and breezy, with soft sand and crashing waves. After a few minutes, tell them to open their eyes and imagine they are riding bikes to the beach. Still lying on their backs, have the children lift their legs into the air and move them as if they were

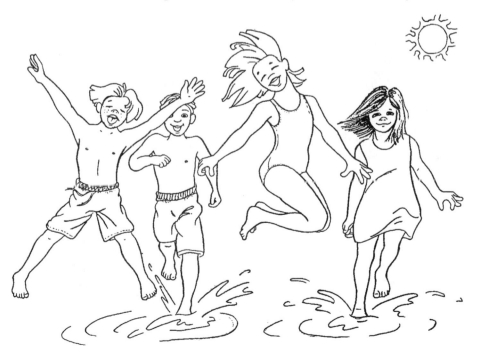

pedaling a bicycle. After a minute, have them reverse the motion, as if they were riding a bicycle backwards.

After about 2 minutes of bicycle pedaling on the floor, ask the children to stand up. Tell them they have not arrived at the beach yet, and they should keep pedaling. Show them how to pedal an imaginary bike by raising their knees one by one and holding imaginary handlebars. The children can ride their imaginary bikes around the room until they reach the beach. Tell them the story below and demonstrate the movements that go with it. Encourage all the children to join in and do the exercises with you.

We stop at the red light and breathe in deeply. When the light changes to green, we start riding again. When we get to the beach, we get off our bikes and lock them. I'll collect the keys on a string so they don't get lost in the sand.

We are tired from all that cycling and need to stretch out. We do this by standing on our tiptoes and swinging our arms above our heads two or three times.

First we walk through the deep sand. The sand is hard to walk through, so take slow, heavy steps. Soon the sand becomes firmer and we can walk normally. We find a good spot on the sand, spread out our towels, and sit down.

Before children get into the "water," have a 10-minute discussion about who can swim, who enjoys the water, and who does not—and why. Many children are afraid of deep water, jellyfish and other sea creatures, being knocked over by waves, putting their heads underwater, being splashed by other children. Discuss these fears in the group. If children are afraid of water, you might tell them the following:

Being afraid is not bad. Sometimes it can be very sensible, because the sea can be dangerous—fear can help keep you from going out too far, for instance. But if your fears keep you from playing in the waves, you will miss out on a lot of fun. It is easier to try it with friends. You can feel brave together. How can you help each other? What could you do to help each other feel safer?

Children might suggest ideas such as: Never swim alone, go into the water gradually (or jump in all at once, depending on their style), don't splash each other, don't go in too deep, let someone who is not afraid go in front of you, hold hands with someone. Tell them that they will have the chance to try out these solutions right now. Stretch a rope along the floor and tell the children that it shows the water's edge. On the other side of that rope are the crashing waves.

Tell the children they wore their bathing suits under their clothes. Invite them to pretend to get undressed down to their bathing suits and put on goggles, snorkel and mask, swim fins, or anything else they like to wear in the water. When they are ready, they should wade in or jump in.

Guide the children in pretending to play in the waves. Tell them when big waves are coming, and invite them to jump over the waves on their own. Then ask the children to line up along the water line and hold hands. Invite the group to try jumping over waves all together. This is harder than it sounds. The children need to coordinate their efforts so they don't pull each other over. Giving a clear rhythm can help a lot. Through playing and talking, all the situations the children found scary can be acted out, along with solutions. This part of the game takes about 10 minutes.

All that playing in the waves can get tiring, so let the children flop down on their bellies or their backs and warm themselves in the sunshine. Tell them:

The sun helps you to relax and you feel very heavy. Your breathing gets deeper and deeper. Far away you hear the waves and the sound of seagulls.

Let them rest like this for about 5 minutes. Then ask them to stretch out and slowly stand up again. Lead them in pretending to get dressed and get back on the bikes. Once again, have them pedal their imaginary bikes around the room by picking up their knees one by one. When you reach home, invite everyone to sit in a circle and talk about the great time they had at the beach.

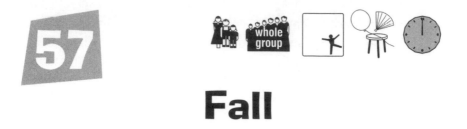

57

Fall

Props: autumn leaves; acorns, maple "propellers," or other autumn "litter"; edible nuts (optional)

♪ **Music:** "Autumn" from *The Four Seasons* by Antonio Vivaldi

Fall is a feast for the senses. The leaves turn such wonderful colors, and the woods smell of damp earth. Leaves, acorns, horse chestnuts, and maple "propellers" have been blown from the trees. The breathing exercises in this lesson require children to let go, just as the trees have let go of their leaves. We are able to let go only when we feel stable and secure. Children initially find security in their parents, but later a child needs to develop his own strength and stability. The "tree stretches" in this lesson help children to stand firm and tall. Developing a firm stance can help children learn to stand on their own two feet in a figurative sense. Contact with the earth is very important.

Have the children spread out around the room. You might begin by explaining the lesson instructions as follows:

Have you ever walked through deep piles of fallen leaves, scuffing your feet and kicking leaves into the air? Let's start with that. Stay on the spot and kick first with one foot, then with the other, as if you were kicking leaves. Now walk around the room, kicking the leaves away.

Kicking will make the children more aware of their feet. This is an excellent preparation for the tree exercise that emphasizes contact with the ground. The children should find themselves a comfortable place and pretend to become a tree. You might guide them as follows:

Let your feet grow like roots into the ground. It is autumn and the trees are bare. Bring your arms up as you breathe in and keep them up as you exhale. Your arms become branches. Your feet stay still on the ground. Let your branches sway back and forth a little in the wind.

From here, lead the children into the following balancing exercise:

Now we do the same thing, but you stand as tall as you can on tiptoes. Move your branches back and forth. Balance for a minute, then come back down from your toes.

Now the tree lets its branches hang down and we bend over to the front and hang there for a moment, coming up again as you exhale.

Repeat the forward bend exercise three times. Then ask the children to sit down for a meditation (sitting still) exercise. Put a leaf on the ground in front of each child. Tell them:

Look carefully at your leaf. Take it into your hand and look at the shape, the color, the texture. When you have looked at it for a while, put it down in front of you and close your eyes. Try to keep the leaf in your mind's eye. We will be very quiet for this exercise.

After a few minutes, ask them to open their eyes again and tell everyone their thoughts and feelings.

Put out leaves, acorns, and other autumn "litter" on the floor. The children walk around to the music. Tell them that whenever the

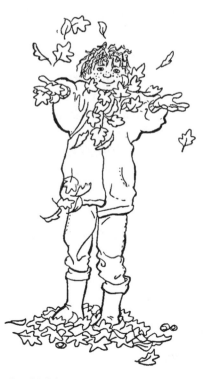

music stops, they should pick up the closest leaf or nut. When the music starts again, they should put the object down and move on.

You can make this into a contact game by letting the children pick something up and swap objects with someone else when the music stops. There are plenty more variations you can think of, or the children can come up with their own ideas.

Next come the breathing exercises. See game 5 on page 22 (Blowing Leaves) for more ideas and information. Seat the children in a circle and place the leaves in the center. Have each child hold a leaf in her hand and blow on it gently. Then invite the children to throw the leaves into the air and blow them into the center of the circle.

Ask the children to lie on their bellies facing the center of the circle. Invite them to imagine they are strong storm winds, and blow hard at the leaves all at once. The leaves will lift from the ground a little. The children will automatically rest their heads on their right and left cheeks in order to blow harder. Some may lift their heads up. It's quite a challenge to make the leaves dance. Through this game they will find different ways of using the breath—hard and soft, short and long—while they stay on their bellies.

Have the children sit again in their circle and give them each an acorn. Tell them:

Put the acorn in front of your right foot. Pick it up with the toes of your right foot and put it down in front of your left foot. Now try to do the same thing with your left foot. (Do this about five times.)

Now that you've got the hang of it, we're going to have some fun. Still using your toes, pass your acorn to the person on your left. Keep passing the acorns around the circle until I tell you to stop.

Let the children keep the acorns. Players might enjoy nibbling on roasted nuts such as pecans or cashews as you discuss the lesson together at the end of class. (Make sure in advance that none of the children are allergic to nuts.)

58

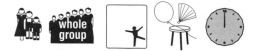 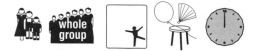

Winter

Props: mats

♪ **Music:** music for ice skating; relaxing music

Whether the winter season in your area is rainy, snowy, or just a little cooler, winter often means children spend more time indoors. They can become quite restless. This lesson lets them imagine playing outside in a winter wonderland. The winter setting provides a good excuse for introducing "hah" breathing and for practicing some dynamic movements borrowed from skating exercises.

Have the children find a place to lie down. If it snows in your area, invite children to imagine that today is a "snow day"—school has been called off because of icy roads. If not, invite them to imagine they are visiting the North Pole. Tell them:

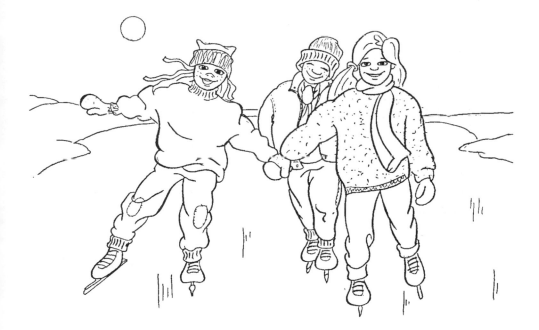

You are still in your nice warm bed. Think about what games you would like to play outside in the snow. Now stretch out and stand up. Make a sideways sweeping movement to open the curtains. Stretch your arms up over your head and down to your sides again.

It's so cold outside that the window is covered with white frost. Open your mouth and breathe "hah" against the glass to melt the frost with your warm breath. Now you can see through the window. Everything is blanketed with snow.

Now we really want to go outside, so we wash quickly (mime washing) *and get dressed* (mime dressing). *Put on your sweater: First raise the left arm, then the right arm, then bring your arms down and let the sweater drop over your head. Put your pants on: First raise your left knee, then lower it into the left pants leg, then raise your right knee and lower it.*

Take your time with this part of the lesson. Children like to dress properly with all the zippers and buttons. Don't forget coat, scarf, gloves, boots, and hat, but don't let it go on *too* long. (Five minutes should be enough.)

Tell the children that everyone will walk through the snow to a small pond that has frozen solid. You're going to go skating. When you reach the ice, lead them in some skating warm-ups. Explain that these are real skating exercises:

Stand up straight with your arms out to the side. Bend forward with a flat back and turn your body so that your right hand touches your left foot and your left hand goes up into the air. Turn your head to look up at your left hand. Now turn your body the other way, so that your left hand touches your right foot and your right hand goes up into the air. Keep switching sides. Once you have the hang of it, try moving faster and faster.

Now we'll do a balancing exercise. Stand on your left foot and bend your right knee so that your right foot rises up behind you. Stretch your right hand back and grab your foot. Hold your right foot in your right hand for the count of two. Now hold the left foot with the left hand.

Next, cross your left foot over your right foot. Walk around the room for a minute, keeping your legs crossed. Now switch legs: Cross your right over your left. Walk around the room again.

Now invite the children to lace up their skates and go out onto the ice. If you like, play music to inspire the movement. If you are playing on a smooth, slippery floor, you might have the children slide across the floor in their socks. If the floor is not slippery, the children might step around the room imitating the movements of speed skaters: They can take long strides, cross their feet over, and swing their arms from side to side.

You might place a pile of mats in the middle of the floor and tell the children it is a rock or fallen tree rising out of the ice. Invite them to skate up to the mats and climb over on hands and knees to the other side.

After the children have experimented with "skating" solo for a while, have them form pairs and skate on together, holding hands. Help them coordinate their movements by giving them a signal for everyone to start skating on the right foot. Let them skate for about 15 minutes total. Then tell them:

It's getting cold now, so we're going to stop skating and go home. To warm yourself up, swing your arms in and out, wrapping them around your body and swinging them loose again. Do this a few times. Now we will trudge home through the snow. Here we are at home; let's sit down in a circle and rub our hands together. Feel the warmth and energy between your hands. Now try it with a partner. Rub your feet together for warmth as well.

Finally, the children can lie down and relax with eyes closed. Play them some relaxing music.

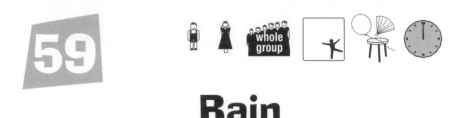

Rain

Props: inflated balloons with a few grains of rice inside

Most adults dislike rain because it is wet, cold, and inconvenient. Children often have more freedom to enjoy the pleasures of rain: puddles for splashing, squishy mud, the feel of raindrops on their face, and the sound of a downpour on the roof. This lesson focuses on the positive aspects of rain—both its pleasures and its benefits.

In the Spring

Music: D. Bersma

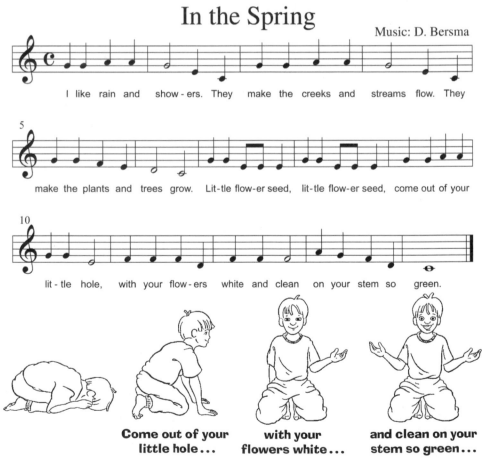

I like rain and show-ers. They make the creeks and streams flow. They make the plants and trees grow. Lit-tle flow-er seed, lit-tle flow-er seed, come out of your lit-tle hole, with your flow-ers white and clean on your stem so green.

Come out of your little hole...　　**with your flowers white...**　　**and clean on your stem so green...**

Begin the class by teaching the children this song, along with the movements shown at the bottom of page 114.

Hand out the balloons and show children how to shake the balloons so that the rice grains make a sound like rain. Invite them to take their balloons and move around the room one by one (or in pairs if you have a large group). Encourage each child or pair to dance, jumping and turning and shaking their balloons to make the sound of rain. Then ask everyone to dance together—they will create a noisy downpour! With a group of older children, you can ask them to pay attention to the rhythm of the rain. For example, you can have one person set a rhythm and ask the others to join in.

Tell the children that it has been raining for a while, and now there are puddles all over the ground. Encourage them to jump and splash in the puddles. Perhaps they can use the balloons to make splashing sounds. Let them all stomp and hop for a while. Then invite them to take turns running up and jumping into a big "puddle" in the middle of the room. The children can let themselves go and will experience a feeling of strength. This is a real grounding exercise—it helps children feel contact with the earth.

Now ask the children to put their balloons aside. Tell them:

Imagine you are a fluffy cloud. When you look at clouds, you can sometimes see funny pictures. A cloud might look like a sheep or a face. Your cloud can be any shape you want. Make a nice shape and move around the room as a cloud, slowly drifting across the sky.

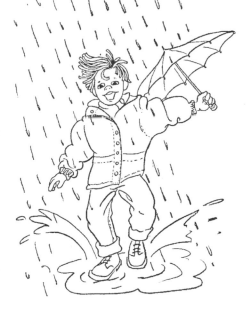

Alternatively, you could have the children form clouds in pairs. After children have a chance to make their own clouds, gather them all together to form one great big storm cloud. Have the group cloud move around the room for a while, then suddenly burst into lots of individual raindrops. Let them bounce around the room as raindrops for a while.

Gather the children into a circle and explain that you will demonstrate a rain massage. Tell them:

Who wants to lie on the ground and feel the rain? Justin, lie on your belly. Everyone else kneel down around him. Justin, we're going to make rain. The special thing about this rain is that you can say where you want to feel it. You can also say if you want it to rain harder or softer. Who wants to help me be the rain? Jessica, Nico, Eli, and I will be the rain.

Put your hands gently on Justin's back, arms, and legs. Can you see where his body moves when he breathes? (Give the children a moment or two to get used to each other.) *Now softly patter your fingertips like raindrops. Justin, you tell us whether you want the rain to fall harder or softer. You can also tell us where you want to feel it.*

Limit the massage to the legs, arms, and back with young children. With older children the rain can fall gently on the head or cheeks.

Once the demonstration is over, form groups of about five players to take turns giving each other rain massages. The person being rained on needs to concentrate on feeling the rain, and the children who are being the rain must listen well to her instructions. The feeling of trust felt by the children that their wishes will be followed is essential to the success of this exercise. After a few minutes the children switch over so that everyone has a chance to feel the rain. Ask them:

As a closing, ask the children how they experienced this massage. Ask them:

How was it? Was it scary? Was it nice? Did the other children listen to what you wanted?

Make sure there is time for all the children to discuss their experiences. Most children enjoy this game very much and ask to do it over and over.

Note: Be sure to check on and follow your school or organization's policies on touching before introducing the massage exercise.

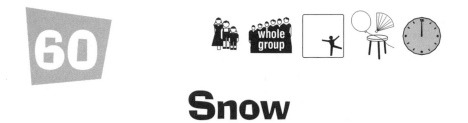

Snow

Props: a cotton ball for each child, an ice cube for each child, one white balloon

The theme of the snow lesson is the experience of the senses: tasting, feeling, listening, looking, and smelling. Snow is a great subject for this, because it changes the outside world so dramatically. Everything looks, feels, sounds, and smells different in the

Snowflakes

Music: D. Bersma

Guess what I saw drift-ing down: snow is fall-ing on our town. Ti-ny
I get up and go out-side but the world is all a-sleep. A white

flakes so white and cold; snow means more to me than gold. Ti-ny
blan-ket helps it hide, snug-gling safe in snow so deep. A white

flakes so white and cold; snow means more to me than gold.
blan-ket helps it hide, snug-gling safe in snow so deep.

A thou-sand thou-sand thou-sand more and more, each flake dif-ferent than be-fore.

Ti-ny flakes so white and cold; snow means more to me than gold.

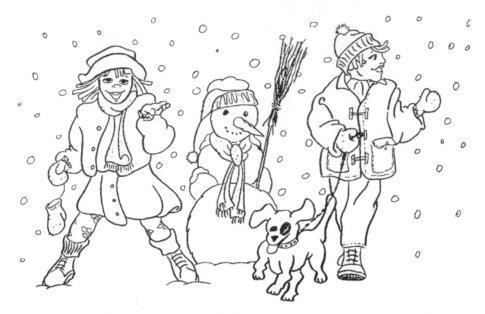

snow. In addition, snow itself is always changing: It can be soft or hard, crisp or slushy, gentle or blinding.

Start by teaching children the song. First read the words aloud twice, then sing the song and let the children join in. You can sing the song several times during the lesson, either with the children or on your own.

Invite the children to move to the song. The song begins with a waltz rhythm. Children might enjoy dancing to this part with a rocking motion. This is interrupted by the 2/4 rhythm at "A thousand...," perfect for marching. The children can also clap to this section. Then the song returns to the waltz rhythm. The children can improvise their own movements to accompany the song.

Now invite the children to imagine that they are out walking in the street when it starts to snow. Suggest that they stand still for a moment and look up at the snow. You can repeat the walking, standing still, and looking up processes two or three times.

The next time children pause, ask them to stand on tiptoes, raise their arms a few times, and catch the snow. This exercise can be quite dynamic, if you encourage the children to move smoothly and quickly, and to bend their knees as they bring their arms down. You can easily combine this exercise with the song above.

Have children walk a little more, then pause again. Ask if they have ever caught snowflakes on their tongues. Invite them to stick out their tongues and taste the snow. Place a small ice cube on each child's tongue. Have them sit down as they suck on the ice cubes. This is an exercise that everyone thoroughly enjoys. When the ice cubes are gone, continue with the following:

Now the ground is completely covered with snow. Walk on your tiptoes and feel how soft the snow is to walk in. See how quietly you can walk.

One by one, have each child come stand by you and listen for the sound of footsteps in the snow. Then gather everyone into a circle. Tell them:

Sit down in the snow, bend forward, and push the snow with your hands toward the center. Together you can build a snow mountain. Make it as tall as you can, but stay sitting. Now sit quietly and think about snow. Put your hands on your belly—what can you feel? Does your belly move as you breathe?

Now ask the children to sit with their legs crossed and hold out their hands. Tell them you will give them each a snowball, and place a cotton ball in each child's hand. Guide them in a breathing exercise—the cotton helps make the breath visible. Tell them:

Blow on the snowflake very softly, so softly that the snowball stays on your hand. Now blow harder and make it fall onto the floor. Pick your snowballs up. Now we'll go around the circle and blow our snowballs off again, one by one.

Continue with body exercises. Now tell them:

Imagine you are a snowball. Lie down and pull your knees up to your belly. Now roll on your back like a snowball. Rock backward and forward and from side to side.

Next, have the children stand in a line and hold hands. Ask the child at one end to stand still as the others circle around her, winding up the line into a tighter and tighter coil. As they wrap themselves up, say "The snowman is getting fatter and fatter!" Say, "The snowman is getting thinner and thinner" to signal them to turn in the other direction, unrolling the line again. Every child will want a turn as the snowman!

Now gather the children into a circle again. Blow up the white balloon and tell them it is a freezing cold snowball. Tell them you are going to pass it around the circle, but everyone must pass it quickly, since it is so cold. (This is a winter version of "hot potato.")

To finish the class, invite the children to lie down in a circle. Sing the song one more time while they relax.

This lesson includes more exercises than some of the others. You might decide to pick and choose from among the exercises, or keep each exercise short and try them all.

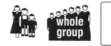

The Balloon's Journey

Props: a blank index card for each child; color pencils in many different colors—enough sets for all the children to make pictures at once; a cotton ball for each child; one ping-pong ball

♪ **Music:** lively selections from Béla Bartók's *For Children*

Humans have always been fascinated with flight. We are bound to the earth, held down by gravity, but our dreams soar with the birds. In this lesson, children send their thoughts and feelings skyward: They imagine attaching a message to a balloon and letting it go. Who knows where it will end up? The lesson also involves movement, color visualization, breathing exercises, sound exercises, and cooperation exercises. We finish with a relaxation exercise.

Begin the lesson with movements to music. Ask the children to skip around the room as the music plays. Tell them that when they hear the music stop, they should freeze in whatever position they are in. While children freeze for a moment, encourage them to notice all the different positions in which the other players are frozen. Start and stop the music several times.

As you play the music for the last time, tell the children that the next time they freeze, they should make a happy sound, such as *hey! wow! whoopee!* Ask them to make a nonsense sound, not say a real word. Then freeze them and listen to the chorus of sounds.

Now ask the children to sit down. Tell them:

Because of the music and the happy sounds, you might be feeling happy. If not, that's okay. You are going to have a chance to tell everyone about how you feel. I'm going to give you all cards upon which you can write about your feelings or draw pictures showing how you

feel. We will attach those cards to imaginary balloons. We will let the balloons go and they will carry our drawings and words away.

First we'll blow up the balloons. Try to imagine that you have a small, limp balloon and choose a color for it. Put the end in your mouth and start to blow it up, slowly and strongly. Blow the imaginary balloon up as big as you like. Tie the end tightly with a string and tie the string to your wrist, a tree, a chair, or whatever you like.

When all the imaginary balloons are inflated and safely tied up, give each child a card and color pencils. Give the children 5 to 7 minutes to make their cards. As children finish their cards, pretend to tie each child's card to the string of her balloon. Then put the cards in a pile for later. Have the children stand together, pretending to hold their balloons. Tell them:

Everyone hold the string of your balloon and make sure your message is attached. Now let go of the string and let your balloon fly up into the air! It floats higher and higher, drifting on the wind. Stand on tiptoes, stretch out as if you're trying to catch it again. But no, it's too

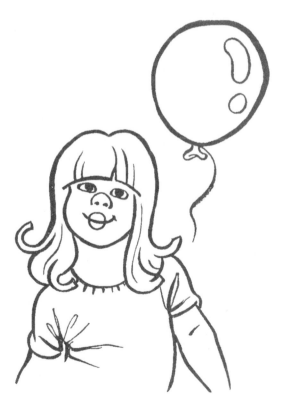

high now. The balloon gets smaller and smaller as it rises until it's just a tiny spot in the sky. The balloon floats away and takes your message with it.

Gather the children into a circle and have them all lie down on their bellies, facing the center. Lie down with them and place a ping-pong ball in front of you. Tell them:

Let's pretend this ping-pong ball is a balloon, and we are breezes blowing it one way and another. We can't touch the ball with our hands: We can only move it with our breath. I'm going to try to blow the ping-pong ball to you, Yvonne. Now you say who you want to pass it to, and blow it that way.

One by one the children call out the names of the people they want to send the ball to. Everyone must get a turn. Then ask the children to lie down on their backs. Tell them:

Pull your knees up and rock back and forth. While you are rocking, think about where your balloon might be.

Straighten out your legs again and lie on your back, or turn on your belly. We're going to tighten up every muscle in our bodies and then let go again. Do that once more. Try to relax completely.

The balloon with your message or drawing has gone far, far away. It is drifting in the air with the sun shining on it. Maybe it's floating over fields, or over trees, or over the mountains, or over the ocean.

Feel your feet, your legs, your belly, your chest, your back, and your face. You are feeling very warm and relaxed. Think about where you would like your balloon to come down and who you would like to read your message or see your drawing.

After a few minutes of quiet relaxation, tell them:

Now come back to the room, feel the floor under you, stretch out, and have a good yawn. Sit up when you're ready.

Ask the children who they think is going to get their message. Spread the cards out on the ground and ask who made them, if they are unsigned. Say something good about each card and ask if you can keep them or if the children want them back. You may learn things about some of the children from their cards. If so, try to include your discoveries in some way in the next lesson.

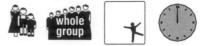

Animals

Children have widely varying temperaments. Some children are shy or fearful; others act tough or make jokes all the time. In this lesson children role-play animals in order to discover that they are not only shy or tough or silly. They can experience a variety of feelings, but those feelings are not who they are. Playing animal characters, children can act out behaviors and consider alternatives. Animals work well for role-play with children. Because it is so obvious that the children are not really lions, birds, or horses, there is no chance that children will confuse fantasy with reality.

Gather the children into a circle and tell them:

Today you can choose an animal that you'd like to be. If you like to be tough and strong, choose an animal you think is like that. If you'd love to fly, choose a bird that lets you feel free. Lie down in a comfortable position, close your eyes, and try to imagine your animal.

Slowly the sun rises and you wake up. Open your eyes and start to move as your animal would move. Run, jump, fly through the room being your animal. If you would like to curl up in your safe, cozy den for a while, that's okay too. Think about how you feel inside and try to move in the same way.

Give the children about 5 minutes to act out their animals independently. Then say:

When you meet another animal, try to react the way these animals might act if they met in the wild. Would you sniff each other? Would one of you run away? See if you can guess what animal everyone has chosen.

After a few more minutes, have everyone sit in a circle again. Ask the children what animals they chose and what it was like to imitate those animals. Then go around the circle and ask each child to act out their animal for everyone to see. When necessary, give individ-

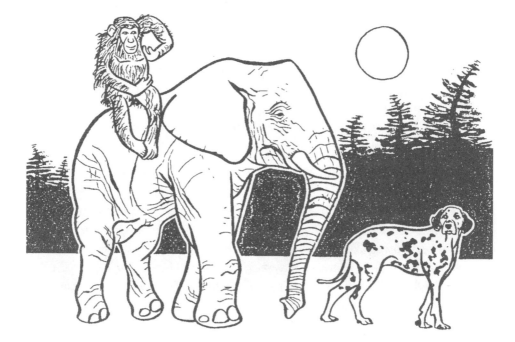

uals some extra ideas and encouragement. Compliment them on their creativity and discoveries. Ask the children what their animals are like: strong, cute, silly.... Ask whether acting those animals made them feel strong, cute, silly, or whatever. After each solo demonstration, invite the rest of the group to imitate that animal. As children try out various animals, they may discover different feelings and characteristics that that animal represents for them. Invite the children to share their thoughts about each animal.

Now invite the children to spread out around the room and choose new animals. Encourage them to choose animals that are very different from the ones they played at first. Imitating other children's animals may have given them new ideas. If they want to play the same animal again, that is okay, too.

This time, guide the children through a more detailed portrayal. Create and tell a story about the animals that includes lots of specific activities. Perhaps they feel hungry and begin looking for food. What kind of food does each animal eat? What sounds do they make?

They may get tired from all that playing and running around and take a rest. Perhaps it will start raining and they have to find shelter. When the sun sets, they may go back to their homes—trees, holes, dens, caves, and so on. There are so many possibilities. The important thing is to think through all the actions the story is likely to inspire. If you don't want the children playing at hunting and killing other animals, don't tell lions to search for food.

End the story with the children lying down. Talk about the different feelings that the animals may display. Tell them:

A particular animal usually acts pretty much the same way: Rabbits are always timid, and bears are always tough and strong. People, on the other hand, may feel very different ways at different times. Sometimes we may feel like a strong lion, sometimes we may feel free as a bird flying through the sky, sometimes we may feel like a silly monkey, and sometimes we may feel like a scared little mouse. You can feel those feelings without being those feelings. Feeling scared doesn't mean that you will always be a scared little mouse.

To end the class, you may want to tell a story that illustrates the idea that you can feel emotions without *being* those emotions. Hans Christian Andersen's "The Ugly Duckling" would work well, or you could make up your own story.

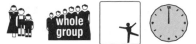

Learning to Fly

Every situation has its positive and negative aspects. Sometimes we see only one side and sometimes only the other. The pros and cons seem to be in opposition but they may actually complement each other. This lesson helps children understand that we can't have the good without the bad. What seems like a disadvantage can later come to seem like an advantage, and vice versa. This lesson uses a baby bird as an example. The nest is cozy and safe, but small and confining as well. Flying offers freedom and excitement, but also danger. Children come to understand the pros and cons in each situation—the bird cannot win freedom without sacrificing security. The lesson also includes breathing exercises and closes with relaxation.

When the children come in, ask them to find a place to sit down. Tell them:

Today we are going to imagine that we are baby birds. The baby birds live together in a warm, cozy nest. Your mother and father bird take good care of you and bring you food. The nest is well hidden in the leaves and feels very safe. Try to imagine this warm, safe feeling.

Remain silent for a minute so that the children have the time to picture the situation. Tell them:

Although you are happy where you are, you begin to get curious about what goes on outside the nest. Now and then you look over the edge of the nest and see all these wonderful things: other trees, other animals, beautiful flowers. They are far away, too far to see them well, but you can smell them just a little bit. Try to imagine the lovely smell of the flowers. Take a slow, deep breath through your nose.

Give the children a couple of minutes to do this breathing exercise. Ask them what they can smell. Then tell them:

Because your parents love you and bring you such good food, you are growing bigger. The nest is starting to feel small and you want more space. You feel your wings growing and you try to open them a bit. You get to the edge of the nest and flap your wings a bit.

Show the children how to flap their arms up and down like baby birds learning to fly. Give them a couple of minutes to practice. Then tell them:

You really want to know what the flowers you smelled look like. You want to meet other birds and you are very curious to know what else there is out there. You want to fly through the air, but at the same time you are a little bit scared. You don't know what is out there in the world. There might be a hawk or a cat waiting to catch you. But still you want to fly free. When you pluck up the courage, jump from the nest and fly around the room. If you get tired, you can go back to your nest, but you can also take a rest on a branch in another tree. Try it.

The children should flap their arms up and down as they walk or run around the room. Join in and, if necessary, encourage the little ones to fly. Now and then they can rest in their starting place (the nest) or somewhere else (an imaginary branch). Older children can choose when they want to fly and when they want to take a rest. With younger children you may want to use a handclap to signal them that it's time to switch from flying to resting, or vice versa.

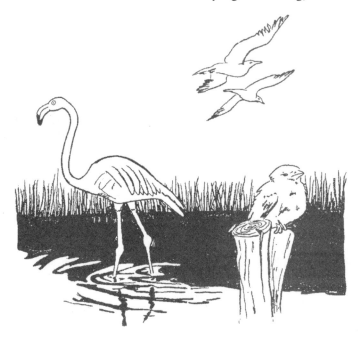

After about 10 minutes, ask the children to find a spot and sit down. Continue the story:

The birds are so happy that they want to sing. Squeeze your mouth up into a little, tight circle. Put your hand on your belly so you can feel how it moves. Hold your other hand a few inches in front of your mouth and feel the air as you blow it out. Now try to make a sound as you do this. First very softly. . . . (after a minute) *and now harder.*

Let children practice whistling for about 5 minutes total. Younger children may need to devote a great deal of concentration to this exercise, or they can merely chirp. You may want to increase older children's awareness of the vocal muscles by drawing their attention to what is happening inside to produce the sound. The children must tighten the belly muscles to force the air out. They can feel this happening because they feel the belly muscles move with one hand as they feel the breath on the other. The face and mouth muscles are used in order to whistle. They are exhaling against slight resistance so the throat relaxes, bringing a feeling of space into the throat. Remind children to breathe in when they need to; if they feel dizzy, they should stop whistling and breathe normally. When the children are done whistling, tell them:

The birds want to fly again. Spread your wings. You are a bit tired now so try to move very slowly as if you are flying in slow motion. Fly around the room as slowly as you can (a couple of minutes). *Now you are so tired that you want to go back to your nest and sleep. Go back to the nest. Settle yourself down comfortably.*

When they are all sitting down, ask the children what it was like to be baby birds and learn to fly. After 5 to 10 minutes of discussion, have them lie down with their eyes closed. Explain the exercise in the form of a story, telling them that every situation has different sides, just as a coin has two sides. The sides are not better or worse than each other, they are both just there. Sometimes you want one, sometimes the other. At times a baby bird may want the safety of the nest, and at other times the bird may want the freedom of flying. Tell them a suitable story, depending on what they experienced and how old the children are. With very young children, stick to the theme of baby birds and tell the story again while they are relaxing (5 to 10 minutes).

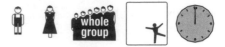

Saying Goodbye

♪ **Music:** lively music

Having a family, friends, and people you care about means sometimes having to say goodbye. Just saying goodbye to their parents at
school in the morning can be hard for young children. Permanent
good-byes are much more difficult. The death of a pet is one
example, but moving to a new town, divorce, and the death of a
grandparent are common experiences for children. They are forced
into a new situation, often without warning. They may feel pain,
anger, denial, and grief.

Saying goodbye is an important part of the process of acceptance, and it is necessary if children are to be able to form new relationships. They need to experience the fact that new relationships
are not replacements, but new and valuable experiences in their
own right. This lesson attempts to help children who have experienced a loss to begin to say goodbye. This sounds like a heavy subject
and, in the case of the loss of a parent or sibling, it may be terrible.
Still, denial and avoidance of the subject are worse. If grief is
hidden, if loss is not accepted, a child will never feel comfortable in
a new situation. If wounds are not given the chance to heal, they will
get in the way of new relationships.

Begin with a simple exercise of making contact and letting go.
Have the children stand in a circle. Don't join the circle yourself—
that way the children will experience contact and letting go solely
with their peers. Ask the children to close their eyes, and tell them:

*Concentrate on your feet and how they feel. Stamp on the ground a
few times. Feel how firmly you are standing.* (After 30 seconds say:)
*Put your hands on your belly and feel the movement of your breath.
Does your belly come out when you breathe in and back again when you*

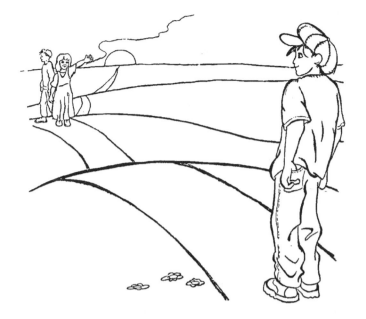

breathe out? (After another 30 seconds say:) *Now let your hands hang by your sides. There are others standing on both sides of you. Keeping your eyes closed, carefully reach your hands out to the sides and hold hands. Notice how their hands feel. Are they warm or cold? Do they feel soft? Are they gripping tightly or loosely? What does your own hand feel like?* (You may want to adapt the exercise for very young children by asking them to open their eyes momentarily when it is time to hold hands. After a couple of minutes say:) *When you are ready, break the contact and let go of each other's hands. Take your time. When your hands are free, you can put them back onto your belly. If you like, you can stamp your feet on the floor again to feel your own feet and your own strength. Open your eyes. What was it like to concentrate on holding hands and letting go?*

After this introduction, guide the children through a movement exercise that involves making contact and letting go. Play music and invite the children to walk around the room. Tell them that when the music stops, they should hold hands with whomever is closest. Challenge them to take hands as fast as they can. The pairs should then sit on the floor. Stop the music and let the children try it. Now tell them that when the music starts again, they should stand up and walk around alone again. Each time the music stops, they should find a different partner. If time allows, keep going until all the children have sat next to each other, hand-in-hand.

Then gather the children into a circle on the ground and read them the following poem:

"Never"

We never named the cat.
We couldn't choose a name, and so we called her Kitty.
She wasn't very friendly, still—
Sometimes she sat on us and rumbled like a truck.
She never said no to a game of tag.
She liked to chase the ghosts of feet under the covers.
We never saw the car that hit her.
My father dug a hole and buried her, alone.
We never said goodbye.

(© 2003 by Ashley Chase)

Afterward, ask the children what they felt about the poem and about their own experiences. Allow plenty of time for this so that the children can express their feelings if they want to. Sadness does not have to be hidden. Letting go plays an important part in the acceptance of change. Talk about how the children let go and made new contacts in the movement exercise. Discuss with children how we can let go and make new contacts in our daily lives.

Finish the lesson with a mirroring exercise (see game 47 on page 91). After such a sad subject, the children will enjoy moving together and feeling each other's support. Have the children stand facing each other in pairs. Tell them to imagine that one partner is looking into a mirror, and the other partner is the image in the mirror. The mirror partner should imitate every move the other partner makes. The children have to observe each other well and follow each other's movements. This requires close cooperation. If the mirror image is not able to follow, the leading child should slow down or choose simpler movements. The children will learn new and different gestures from each other. This exercise is particularly good for stimulating creativity. Make sure the mirror and the other partner switch roles at least once. With this exercise you can also change partners several times. After 5 to 10 minutes, bring this exercise and the lesson to an end.

Field Trip

Props: a long rope, one blindfold for each child (optional)

If the weather is good and there is a park or another open space nearby, it's wonderful to take a class outside. In our daily lives we seldom take the time to enjoy the world outside our door. There are so many sounds we don't hear, fragrances we don't smell, textures we don't feel. You can expand the children's world by making them aware of those sounds, smells, and sensations.

At the park, have the children line up. Extend the rope along the line and ask each child to hold on tight. Explain that you will guide them with the rope, and ask them either to close their eyes or put on blindfolds. Then begin leading the children through the park. Tell them:

Closing your eyes gives you the chance to pay more attention to other senses: hearing, touch, and smell. Be very quiet and listen to all the sounds you can hear. Breathe through your nose: Can you smell anything in the air? As we walk, we may pass trees, flowers, grass, and water. Each of these has its own smell. Try to smell all the different things. We are also going to walk on different surfaces—grass, gravel, concrete. Even through your shoes, the surfaces will feel different: Try to notice them all. I promise not to lead you astray or let you hurt yourselves. Just trust me, and enjoy the walk.

Lead the children past as many different sounds and smells and over as many different surfaces as you can find. You might take them across a lawn, over a bridge, and along a stream. Stop along the way and invite them to feel the texture of rocks, tree bark, and leaves on bushes. When you reach an open lawn suitable for yoga, have them let go of the rope and sit in the grass. Invite each child to tell you what he can hear, feel, and smell right now, or what he remembers from your walk. Ask the children to open their eyes and stand up. Tell them:

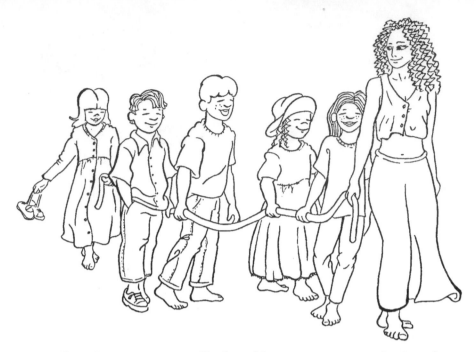

Imagine you are a tree. You have big, strong roots growing into the ground. Take a deep breath. There is a wind and the trees move. The trees can wave their branches in the wind. There are tall trees—make yourself very tall. There are short, wide trees—now get low, stretch out your arms, and make yourself as wide as you can.

Lead the children in the traditional yoga tree pose. You will find a detailed description in game 18 on pages 40–41 (The Tree).

To finish your lesson in the park, lead the children in sun salutations. You will find a detailed description in game 28 on page 60 (Sun Salutations for Children). Then show the children how to walk back the way you came in a meditation walk. Tell them:

Put the heel of one foot against the toes of the other foot. Change feet very consciously. Concentrate on walking and don't talk for now. We will walk part of the way back like this.

After a few minutes, invite the children to begin walking normally again. Lead them back to the room. When you return, if time allows, ask the children to lie on their mats for a few minutes. Discuss your journey through the park and the senses everyone used.

66

The Body

Props: mats, a large sheet of paper, a thick magic marker, colored markers or crayons

In the West, we divide the unity of ourselves into body and mind. In fact, they are irrevocably bound to each other. Understanding our bodies and being in good physical shape helps us to be in better shape emotionally and mentally. We can exercise the body to help prepare us to use our minds. We may warm up our voices before giving a speech, stretch out our hands to help us write or type, and count on our fingers when working out math problems. Being in tune with our bodies helps us to concentrate, deal better with our emotions, and be flexible when encountering the unexpected.

Place the paper on the floor and invite a volunteer to lie down on it. Use the marker to trace around the volunteer, leaving the outline of her body on the paper. Have all the children sit in a circle around the drawing. You might instruct them as follows:

*Sit still and move just your **head**. How many different movements can you make? Make the movements gentle. Closing your eyes will help you feel what happens when you move your head. Look to the left, look to the right, and bend your head forward and backward. Then hold it up straight again. On your head is your **hair**. Touch your hair gently with your hands. Feel how long your hair is. Tap your fingertips gently on your head.*

*Now gently feel your **ears** with your fingers. You will feel hard parts and soft parts. Try pulling gently on your earlobes. Move your hands to your **cheeks**. Rub them and pinch them gently. How do they feel? Is there a difference between your right and left cheeks?*

*Can you raise your **eyebrows**? Can you lower them? How does this feel in your forehead? Does it give you wrinkles? Feel your forehead with your hands. Close your **eyes**. Now open them again. Now close*

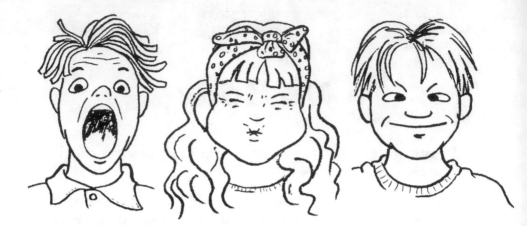

your eyes as tight as you can—scrunch your eyelids up—and then open them, as wide as you can. Now relax your eyes again.

Can you flare your **nostrils**? Try sniffing and then breathing out through your nose.

How can you move your **mouth**? How wide can you open it? Can you click your teeth together? Try to move every part of your mouth you can think of. What can you do with your **tongue**? Run your tongue along your teeth and let it get to know the whole inside of your mouth. Can you stick out your tongue to the left and to the right? Can you roll your tongue into a tube? Can you make it flat? How do you look when you're **happy** or **sad**? When you are **angry** or **surprised**? Can you make **funny faces**?

Invite the children to use the colored markers or crayons to fill in and label all the different parts of the head on the body outline you traced. Then tell them:

Now stand up and spread the circle out a little. While standing in one place, how many ways can you move your **body (torso)**? Let's try some gentle movements together. We can turn to the left and to the right, we can bend over forwards and backwards, we can bend to the left and to the right. Now stand up straight again.

Swing your **arms** side to side, up and down, around in circles. Shrug your **shoulders** up and down, and turn them in circles, forward and back. Bend and unbend your **elbows**. Bend your **wrists** up and down, and then twirl them gently in circles. Now shake out your arms and hold your **hands** in front of you. How many different movements can you make with your **fingers**? How fast can you wiggle them? Can you bend and stretch them one by one? Are there some fingers that can't move alone? Try every movement you can think of.

Have the children label the parts of the arms and hands on the body outline and tell them:

Now lie down on the floor on your backs. Feel your **heart**. How is it beating? How does your **belly (abdomen)** feel? When you put your hands on your belly, do you feel your breath moving there, or do you feel your breath somewhere else in your body? Put your hands on the **left** and **right** sides of your body. What do they feel like?

Now concentrate on your **back**. Is your back relaxed on the ground? Can you feel where your back is touching the ground and where there is a space? When you breathe in, does the shape of your back on the floor get bigger? Can you feel where your **shoulders** are touching the ground? Can you feel where each **vertebra** in your spine touches the ground? Can you feel your **bottom** on the ground?

Now children can fill in on the outline the body parts you just discussed. Then tell them:

Stand up and spread out. Let's see all the things you can do with your **legs** while staying in one place. You can do lots of things, can't you? You can walk on the spot, stand on tiptoes, or stamp your **feet** on the ground. You can swivel your **hips** from side to side or around in a circle. You can bend your **knees**. You can shake your right leg or your left leg. You can kick your legs up in the air.

Sit down again and see what you can do with your legs while you're sitting. Can you move them differently? Try pointing your feet and flexing them back toward you. Try bending your **ankles** from side to side, and then twirling them in circles. What can you do with your **toes**?

Have the children finish filling in the body outline. Then lead them in a relaxation exercise. Tell them:

We have just discovered lots of things we can do with our bodies. Another thing we can do is tense our bodies and relax them. We are going to finish this lesson by relaxing. Find yourself a nice spot. When you are lying comfortably on your back, we'll continue. While you breathe in deeply, tense up all the muscles in your body from head to *toe. Stay like that a moment, then breathe out through your mouth and relax all your muscles again. One more time: Tense your body, then relax. Your whole body should now feel warm and very relaxed. Stay like that for a while.*

After 5 minutes, ask the children to stand up slowly. You can then invite the volunteer whose body you traced to take the drawing home with her.

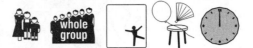

Birthday Party

Props: cupcakes or other treats brought in by the birthday child; mats

Birthdays are special days for children. Children often want to give their friends a treat—even in yoga class. It is very easy to gobble down treats and wish for more, without ever pausing to appreciate their color, scent, taste, or texture. This lesson helps children savor a treat. It also uses various activities to explore the idea of giving and receiving.

Begin the lesson by singing "Happy Birthday" to the birthday child. Sing it in the usual way first, then have the children spread out and show them movements to add:

- "Happy birthday to you"—*we bring our arms above our heads and get as tall as we can*

- "Happy birthday to you"—*we open our arms wide and get as broad as we can*

- "Happy birthday, dear Paco"—*we put both hands on our hearts*

- "Happy birthday to you!"—*we put our hands out, palms up in a giving gesture*

Explain that the birthday child has brought treats for everyone. Show the treats, and then have the birthday child pass the treats out to everyone in the room. Ask the children to wait until you tell them to eat the treats; everyone will eat at the same time. Tell them:

Have a good look at what you have been given. What is its shape and color? Try to imagine how it's going to taste. Take the paper off carefully (if necessary). Lick your treat very gently with your tongue.

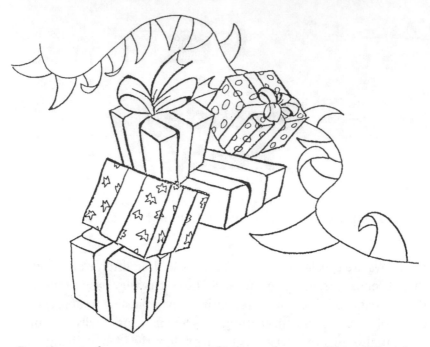

Does it taste the way you imagined? Now take a small bite. What does it feel like? Is it crunchy or creamy? Is it good to chew? As you eat your treat, think about how it looks, smells, tastes, and feels.

If the treat is not edible, but something else like a small toy or party favor, ask the children to imagine what they are going to do with it. Have them tell their plans to the class one by one. It is great for the children when their treats are taken so seriously.

Afterward, let the birthday child choose some yoga games for everyone to do. Game 23 on pages 51–52 (Back Roll, Rag Doll, and Plow) would be a good birthday game, since kids make the shape of a birthday cake with candles by lying in a circle with their legs in the air. Other fun choices might be: game 3 on pages 19–20 (Airball), game 13 on page 32 (Animal Sounds), game 20 on page 45 (The Frog), game 22 on pages 48–49 (The Cat), game 51 on page 95 (Lean on Me), or game 53 on page 98 (Stick Together).

Here are a few more ideas for birthday games:

- The birthday child walks around the room and the others follow and imitate him. When the birthday child stops, the other children freeze in their last position. The children can hop, skip, crawl on their bellies, or walk on hands and feet. There are endless possibilities. This exercise is exciting and fun because players never know when they might have to freeze.

- Gather all the children around you. Strike a pose and invite the children to imitate you. Challenge the children to follow your lead as you keep changing your position. You can add to the fun and excitement by making changes abruptly, or in quick succession. The children can then take turns leading this game.

About 5 or 10 minutes before the end of class, invite the birthday child to find a spot to sit down. Ask the others to sit in a circle around the birthday child, close their eyes, and think of a wish for him.

After a few moments, invite the children to open their eyes and tell their wishes one by one. Often the children make wishes they also want for themselves. In this exercise children will often reveal quite a lot about themselves. Affirm their feelings and make a mental note to see if there is something you can cover in a subsequent lesson.

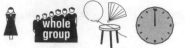

Making Mandalas

Props: large sheets of newsprint (unprinted) or old newspapers; sheets of drawing paper with a large circle drawn on each; markers and pastels or plenty of colored pencils; rulers; examples of mandala forms from nature (for example, flowers and sliced fruit)

♪ **Music:** relaxing music (optional)

Colors influence our emotions. We delight in the colors bouncing from a raindrop. Drawing with colorful markers, crayons, or pencils helps children express feelings they can't always communicate in words.

The word *mandala* comes from the Sanskrit and means "circle" or "center." A mandala is a form with radial symmetry: The circular design is organized regularly around a center point. Mandalas are divided into equal sections, or concentric rings, or a combination of both. Mandalas can be found everywhere in nature. Most flowers have petals radiating from a center. An orange half, a tree stump, a spider web, a starfish, and a snowflake are all mandala forms. So are our own eyes, with the iris surrounding the pupil in the center. Buddhists use the mandala to represent the universe. The circle forms a whole. It holds everything inside itself.

Begin the lesson with a loosening-up drawing. Spread out blank newsprint (or old newspapers), put out markers, and invite the children to doodle. Encourage them to make big, sweeping strokes on the newsprint, tracing figure eights and waves. Stop this warm-up exercise after about 5 minutes.

Discuss mandala designs with the children and display mandala forms from nature, such as flowers or cut fruit. Ask the children to sit down and close their eyes. Tell them:

Imagine that you are standing in the center of a circle. You are the center of the mandala. While you breathe gently, the circle begins to grow bigger. What can you see in the circle? It could be anything. You

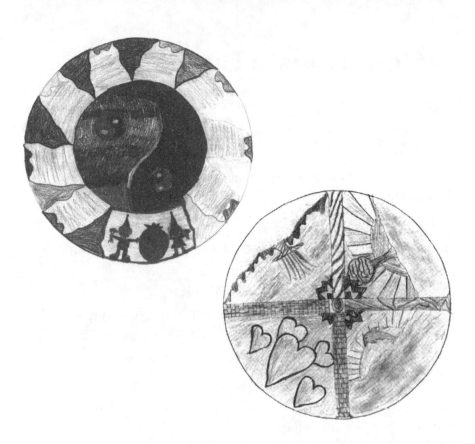

might see abstract designs, or symbols, or things from real life. Look at the colors and the shapes. In a minute we are going to make mandalas, and you can draw and color what you see in your mind now. Your mandalas will be different, but they will all be beautiful.

After about 2 minutes, ask the children to open their eyes again and give them each a sheet of paper with a circle drawn on it. Now they can work with pastels or crayons. If necessary, offer help and encouragement. You might help the children use a ruler as a straightedge to divide the circle into four or more sections, if they like. Remind the children that they can draw whatever they want in their mandalas. Play relaxing music if it will help the children concentrate. When the drawings are finished, display them all and ask each child to talk about her mandala. If some children are not able to finish their mandalas in time, they can take them home or finish them during the next lesson.

Some Music Suggestions

Aeoliah: *The Seven Chakras: Crystal Illumination*

Anugama: *Silent Joy*

Béla Bartók: *For Children*

Ludwig van Beethoven: *Minuets* (suggested for when dancing blindfolded)

Erik Berglund: *Harp of the Healing Waters*

Georges Bizet: *Jeux d'enfants* (suggested for exercises involving rolling around)

Fryderyk Chopin: some quiet Op. 28 Preludes

Edvard Grieg: *Peer Gynt Suite* (suggested for when bouncing like a frog)

Gustav Holst: *The Planets* (suggested for relaxation exercises)

Julian Lloyd Webber: *Lullaby*

Modest Mussorgsky: *Pictures at an Exhibition* (suggested for exercises involving drawing)

Sergey Prokofiev: *Peter and the Wolf* (suggested for when moving like a cat)

Maurice Ravel: *Mother Goose Suite*

Camille Saint Saëns: *Carnival of the Animals* (suggested for relaxation exercises or for when moving like a frog or cat)

Erik Satie: *Early Piano Works*

Robert Schumann: *Carnaval* (suggested for exercises involving drawing)

Pyotr Il'yich Tchaikovsky: *Sleeping Beauty* (suggested for sleeping or relaxation exercises)

Antonio Vivaldi: *The Four Seasons*

Andreas Vollenweider: *Behind the Gardens, Behind the Wall, Under the Tree...*

Andreas Vollenweider: *White Winds*

The Games Arranged According to Age Groups

Preschool—Grade 5
(Ages 3–11)

1. Breathing and Awareness
2. Belly Breathing
3. Airball
5. Blowing Leaves
6. Seeing the Breath
7. Air Volley
8. Feeling the Breath
9. Opening the Throat
10. Breath on the Window
11. Sounds
12. Singing Names
13. Animal Sounds
17. The Mountain
19. Sitting Postures
20. The Frog
21. Lying Down, the Rest Position
22. The Cat
27. Child's Pose
31. Sleep
34. Rag Doll
44. Seeing-Eye Guide
45. Two Guides
49. Jumping Together
55. Spring
56. Summer
57. Fall
58. Winter
60. Snow
61. The Balloon's Journey
62. Animals
63. Learning to Fly
66. The Body
67. Birthday Party

Kindergarten—Grade 2
(Ages 5–8)

4. Air Soccer
14. Side Breathing
18. The Tree
23. Back Roll, Rag Doll, and Plow
24. The Cobra
25. The Grasshopper
26. The Swan
28. Sun Salutations for Children
29. Shake It Loose
30. Being Heavy
33. Energy in Your Hands
35. Tensing and Relaxing
36. What Does Tension Feel Like?
46. Dancing Together
47. The Mirror
48. Walking Backward
51. Lean On Me
52. A Massage
59. Rain
64. Saying Goodbye
65. Field Trip

Kindergarten–Grade 5

(Ages 5–11)

4. Air Soccer
14. Side Breathing
18. The Tree
23. Back Roll, Rag Doll, and Plow
24. The Cobra
25. The Grasshopper
26. The Swan
28. Sun Salutations for Children
29. Shake It Loose
30. Being Heavy
33. Energy in Your Hands
35. Tensing and Relaxing
36. What Does Tension Feel Like?
46. Dancing Together
47. The Mirror
48. Walking Backward
51. Lean on Me
52. A Massage
59. Rain
64. Saying Goodbye
65. Field Trip

Grades 3–5

(Ages 8–11)

4. Air Soccer
14. Side Breathing
15. Back Breathing
16. Feeling Sounds Through the Back
18. The Tree
23. Back Roll, Rag Doll, and Plow
24. The Cobra
25. The Grasshopper
26. The Swan
28. Sun Salutations for Children
29. Shake It Loose
30. Being Heavy
32. White Light
33. Energy in Your Hands
35. Tensing and Relaxing
36. What Does Tension Feel Like?
37. A Space of Your Own
46. Dancing Together
47. The Mirror
48. Walking Backward
50. Circle of Friends
51. Lean on Me
52. A Massage
53. Stick Together
54. Lost and Found
59. Rain
64. Saying Goodbye
65. Field Trip
68. Making Mandalas

SmartFun activity books encourage imagination, social interaction, and self-expression in children. Games are organized by the skills they develop and simple icons indicate appropriate age levels, times of play, and group size. Most games are noncompetitive and require no special skills or training. The series is widely used in homes, schools, day-care centers, clubs, and summer camps.

101 MUSIC GAMES FOR CHILDREN: Fun and Learning with Rhythm and Song *by* Jerry Storms

All you need to play these 101 music games are music tapes or CDs and simple instruments, many of which kids can have fun making from common household items. Many games are especially good for large group settings, such as birthday parties and day care. Others are easily adapted to meet classroom needs. No musical knowledge is required.

Translated into 11 languages worldwide!

160 pages ... 30 illus. ... Paperback $12.95 ... Spiral bound $17.95

101 MORE MUSIC GAMES FOR CHILDREN: New Fun and Learning with Rhythm and Song *by* Jerry Storms

This action-packed compendium offers musical activities that children can play while developing a love for music. Besides listening, concentration, and expression games, this book includes rhythm games, relaxation games, card and board games, and musical projects. **A multicultural section** includes songs and music from Mexico, Turkey, Surinam, Morocco, and the Middle East.

176 pages ... 72 illus. ... Paperback $12.95 ... Spiral bound $17.95

101 DANCE GAMES FOR CHILDREN: Fun and Creativity with Movement *by* Paul Rooyackers

The games in this book combine movement and play in ways that encourage children to interact and express how they feel in creative fantasies and without words. They are organized into meeting and greeting games, cooperation games, story dances, party dances, "musical puzzles," dances with props, and more. No dance training or athletic skills are required.

160 pages ... 30 illus. ... Paperback $12.95 ... Spiral bound $17.95

For more information visit www.hunterhouse.com

101 MORE DANCE GAMES FOR CHILDREN: New Fun and Creativity with Movement *by* Paul Rooyackers
Designed to help children develop spontaneity and cultural awareness, the highly original games in this book include Animal Dances, Painting Dances, Dance Maps, and Dance a Story. The **Dance Projects from Around the World** include Hula dancing, Caribbean Carnival, Maypole, Chinese Dragon Dance, and Brazilian Capoeira.

176 pages ... 48 b/w photos. ... Paperback $12.95 ... Spiral bound $17.95

101 DRAMA GAMES FOR CHILDREN: Fun and Learning with Acting and Make-Believe
by Paul Rooyackers
Drama games are a fun, dynamic form of play that help children explore their imagination and creativity. These noncompetitive games include introduction games, sensory games, pantomime games, story games, sound games, games with masks, games with costumes, and more. The "play-ful" ideas help to develop self-esteem, improvisation, communication, and trust.

160 pages ... 30 illus. ... Paperback $12.95 ... Spiral bound $17.95

101 MORE DRAMA GAMES FOR CHILDREN: New Fun and Learning with Acting and Make-Believe
by Paul Rooyackers
These all-new drama games require no acting skills—just an active imagination. The selection includes morphing games, observation games, dialog games, living video games, and game projects. **A special multicultural section** includes games on Greek drama, African storytelling, Southeast Asian puppetry, Pacific Northwest transformation masks, and Latino folk theater.

144 pages ... 33 illus. ... Paperback $12.95 ... Spiral bound $17.95

101 LANGUAGE GAMES FOR CHILDREN: Fun and Learning with Words, Stories and Poems
by Paul Rooyackers
Language is an essential human skill—perhaps the most important one—and a sense of fun can make our language more creative and memorable. This book contains over one hundred language games and variations that have been tested in classrooms around the world. They

For more information visit www.hunterhouse.com

range from simple letter games and sensory games that teach young children words for sensations and feelings, to more advanced word play, story-writing games, and poetry games including Hidden Word and Haiku Arguments. This book will be an essential tool for English teachers and an inspiration for most parents.

144 pages ... 24 illus. ... Paperback $12.95 ... Spiral bound $17.95

101 MOVEMENT GAMES FOR CHILDREN: Fun and Learning with Playful Movement *by* Huberta Wiertsema

Movement games help children develop sensory awareness, ease and skill of movement, self-condence and daring, and using movement for self-expression.The games are organized in sections including reaction games, cooperation games, and expression games, and include variations on old favorites such as Duck, Duck, Goose as well as new games such as Mirroring, Equal Pacing, and Moving Joints.

160 pages ... 49 illus. ... Paperback $12.95 ... Spiral bound $17.95

YOGA GAMES FOR CHILDREN: Fun and Fitness with Postures, Movements and Breath
by Danielle Bersma and Marjoke Visscher

A playful introduction to yoga for children ages 6–12. The games help young people develop body awareness, physical strength, and flexibility. The 54 exercises are variations on traditional yoga exercises, adjusted for children and clearly illustrated. Ideal for warm-up classes and relaxing time-outs at school or at home.

160 pages ... 69 illus. ... Paperback $12.95 ... Spiral bound $17.95

UPCOMING ... for Ages 6 and up

101 IMPROV GAMES FOR CHILDREN AND ADULTS
by Bob Bedore   *October 2003*

Introducing the next step in drama and play skills: a guide to creating something out of nothing, for reaching people using skills you didn't know you possessed. Contains instructions for teaching improv to children, advanced improv techniques, and tips for thinking on your feet—all from an acknowledged master of the improv form.

For more information visit www.hunterhouse.com